Glutton Free

The Case for Fitness in the 21st Century

-Steve Pavel

Table Of Contents

Introduction

It's 2017. 35.7% of people living in the United States of America are considered obese. In the 1950s, roughly 10% of Americans were obese. In total, 68.8% of Americans are overweight or obese. Trends tell us that by the year 2030, 9 out of 10 Americans will be overweight or obese. As of this writing, I see no evidence of a coming course correction.

Since the 1950s and the rise of fast food, along with the subsequent exponential evolution of technology, our capitalist system has created a climate that facilitates this new age of inactivity, gluttony, and obesity. In generations past, only the wealthy were overweight. Scarcity in food supply is no more, at least in America, as a poor person on food stamps now fills their cart with frozen pizzas, soda, and deep fried twinkies. Obesity and gluttony are rapidly becoming the norm, and any objective observer should see that there isn't much momentum pushing in the other direction. While there is in fact a rise in fresh food markets, and the fitness and nutrition industry is growing by double digits year over year, and the coming generation has even at times been called, "Generation Wellness," an empowered group of young people with information and idealist intentions on their side, I still don't see a course correction anytime soon.

Even with the rise of fresh markets and youthful, idealist based inspiration, there stands a fast food establishment on almost every corner of America's busy streets. Every store you walk into is prepared to sell you candy bars and soda, even if you went in for cough medicine. We stare endlessly and aimlessly into a myriad of devices that have made life easier, but we stare with sedentary eyes as our screens become increasingly populated with advertisements by companies that facilitate the downfall of American wellness. We exist in consumption based economy and prosperity in this system does not come without caustic byproducts. We need to shift directions and a new paradigm will be needed, a culture shift.

Not only do we eat too much, exercise too little, and blame too often, but we seem to glorify this excess of consumption. In 2012, the world largest hamburger was created. It weighed in at 2,014 pounds. It was over 10 feet wide. It had 60 pounds of bacon, 50 pounds of lettuce, 50 pounds of onion, and 40 pounds of cheese. The burger required a crane to flip it over. We have hotdog and pancake eating contests. We have television programs called, "Man V Food", and "My 600-lb. life." We wrap burgers in bacon and tacos in waffles.

Sandwiched between fast food commercials are infomercials with the newest diet pill. Your friend told you that they lost 8 pounds on the paleo diet, only to gain 15 back. Your co-worker insists that you just need to go gluten free. What you need to do, is go Glutton Free. It's not gluten, or processed food even, or that you don't have time to exercise, or that healthy food is too expensive. It's you. It's your habits. It's your tendency to recoil back into complacency and laziness. America doesn't need to be gluten free, America needs to be glutton free.

Chapter 1: The Rise Of Gluttony
(and the fall of physical activity)

glut-ton-y
noun
habitual greed or excess in eating.

Humble Beginnings.

In 1955 McDonald's formed a business partnership with the Coca-Cola Company, and the first fountain soda was born, offered in a 7-ounce cup. Today, you can walk into any gas station or convenience store in America and watch someone walk out with a 128-ounce bucket of carbonated sugar water. Fast food was new and exciting in the 1950s, families were becoming busier and fast food establishments served as a convenient, affordable way to get meals on the go to take home and eat while they watched their new TV. The first McDonald's opened in the 1940s, and by 1958 had sold it's 100 millionth hamburger. The boom was just beginning. As fast food became more popular, the 1950s effectively gave birth to KFC, Dunkin Donuts, Pizza Hut, White Castle, Wendy's, Church's Chicken, Burger King, Dominoes, and many others. Today nearly 50,000 fast food chains populate the cities and streets of America. Not only has the rise of fast food proven to be one of the biggest and most successful innovations in American history, but it stands alone as one of the biggest, time tested pillars of American culture.

While immensely profitable, the economic growth cultivated by the rise of fast food has been mirrored only by the growth of the American waistline. All good things have consequences, and the rise of fast food coupled with the increase of food consumption, improved efficiency in food production, increase in technology that facilitates inactivity and increasingly sedentary jobs, has developed quite the glutton problem for the United States of America.

Competition is the backbone of capitalism, so it should come as no surprise as to why we have soft drink sizes to match our waistlines. Let's say Company A releases a 12-oz. soda, for one dollar. Company B, who had been serving a 7-oz. soda for a dollar, is at a stark disadvantage. They could match Company A and go to a 12-oz. soda, but then they have the same product and they must rely on other products, services, marketing, and location to win the war. Soda has a low wholesale cost, and fountain drink services are cheap to maintain, inventory doesn't take too much room to stock, so what the hell, how about a 16-oz. soda for a dollar. Next thing you know a dollar gets you 24 oz., then 32, then 48, then 64, and the trend continues. Before long it's 2017, America is obese, but luckily, we get a free refill on our 7th fountain drink from the gas station so we can haul in our bucket handled container of doom and refill that thing with hundreds of grams of carbonated, neon green sugar water. Goes well with a Honey Bun and a pack of cigarettes.

In 2014 7-Eleven planned to offer the "X-Gulp", a 150-oz. giant soda. They were going to make sure that the bucket of cola had a nice handle for ease of carrying. Consumers were weary that the soda would be high priced, or even worse, that the soda might not fit in the cup holder. One vigilant soda drinker was cited in an article saying, "I'll just put the damn thing between my legs when I'm on the road!" Wrong answer, America. Now, I know that these are isolated incidents and I don't intend to act like the fringe is the norm, but the norm is bad enough. Let's put this in perspective. As a fitness trainer, it's common to encourage clients to drink half of their body weight in ounces of water, daily. For me, at 195 pounds this is about 92.5 ounces of water per day. Consumed in regular intervals daily, this is not that difficult to achieve, and the rewards are immeasurable. In dealing with clients and prospects, I always ask the person how much water they drink. Statistics that I've written up over recent months are showing that in my samples, less than 30% of people drink anywhere near enough water. Some tell me they hardly drink a glass a day! So, a 200-pound person needs to drink 100 ounces of water daily, which is a cited struggle, but someone can down 128 ounces of soda in a sitting? I know that most people do not drink a 128-ounce soda, but it's common for someone to pick up a 16 to 32-ounce soda at a convenience store or a drive thru daily. Let me inform you now that a 32-ounce Coca-Cola has 91 grams of sugar, which is literally unacceptable for anyone to drink. Maybe a professional athlete can justify that much sugar during or before a competition, but they certainly aren't getting that sugar from soda. Keep in mind, carbohydrates, or sugar, is used in the body for energy, so when you are going to sit on your ass all day at work, and then sit on your ass at home, you don't need all that much sugar. That which you don't use for energy, turns into body fat.

In 2012, when the Center for Consumer Freedom, a non-profit organization (backed by the fast food industry, conveniently) published a full-page ad in the Sunday New York Times against Michael Bloomberg's proposal to ban sugary drinks over 16 ounces, titled, "New Yorkers need a Mayor, not a Nanny." Unintended consequences are a natural byproduct of profit driven capitalism, and while we aim to maximize economic growth, we must keep ourselves accountable. Unfortunately, if you are overweight and drinking a 64-oz. soda, you might need a nanny more than a mayor. Accountability should be the price of freedom. Accountability, however, is not in high supply. We seem to be, however unfortunate, a whiny, narcissistic, over-indulgent society who doesn't like to be told what to do, even if it's for our own good.

By the way, I'm totally fine with a ban on sugary sodas and fatty foods. If I offended you or lost your interest in reading further, too bad. I know that regulating bad food won't do anything, nor am I calling for it. However, in principle, if you can't be personally responsible enough to maintain healthy habits, (as you'll find out in chapter 2, your bad health habits cost the rest of us a tremendous amount of resources), then maybe you should be monitored until you grow up enough to make better choices. Your mother takes away your matches when you're a kid, but now you're a pestilent adult who whines when the government wants to take something away. I'm sure we'd all feel very sorry for you if your 64-oz sodas were taken away, you poor thing.

Trending upward.

Soda obviously isn't the only thing that has increased in size. Since 1960 the American dinner plate has grown by 36%. The average dinner plate now is around 11 or 12 inches, and decades ago measured about 7 to 9 inches. It is said that humans tend to eat about 92% of what they serve themselves, and studies have shown that simply by switching to slightly smaller plates we will consume less so long as the portion isn't too small to send us back for seconds. Human psychology shows also that we tend to fill our plate, regardless of size. Pick up a big dinner plate and plop a small serving of food in the middle. It just doesn't look right, so we'd better add some more. Take that same serving and place it on a smaller plate and it looks like a meal. Research has shown that by switching to a 10-inch plate from a 12-inch plate, that you will eat on average about 22% less calories.

With this I'm reminded of a conversation I had with a friend of mine recently, regarding his trip to the movies with his kids. When grabbing a soda and some popcorn he was reminded by the enterprising cashier that he could up size his drink and his popcorn, for only a dollar more. This is common, and in America we sure love to get more bang for our buck. I mean, what sort of schmuck doesn't know how to spot a deal when he sees one? This happens in every drive thru, gas station, and grocery store in America. Just the other day I went into a speedway gas station, and even though I was wearing an Anytime Fitness polo on my way to work, I was asked by the cashier if I'd like to buy two candy bars, for only $2.50. This sure is a good deal, considering that a single was a much higher unit price. We are often victims to this value baiting, and why I believe that places like Costco unintentionally make us fatter, because when we buy a bigger bag of potato chips, we eat more potato chips. It's just not in our nature to count out 14 chips that make up a serving size. Go big or go home America.

The Slow Death of Fast Food

According to an article by the Ohio Medical Group in July of 2016, fast food restaurants are now serving 50 million customers per day. McDonald's now serves 75 hamburgers every second! The average American now spends about $1,200 a year on fast food, and more than 1 in 3 children eat fast food every day. Even though there has been a noted rise in the fresh food market, NPR reports that fast food consumption hasn't slowed in fifteen years. Here's a fun fact for you, it is said now that 20% of all American meals are eaten in the car. Like George Carlin said, "I eat fast food in the slow lane."

It's important to note that through the FDA, and even the Affordable Care Act, new regulations now force fast food and similar chains to provide the calories and nutritional content for everything they sell. This is vitally important. Just a reminder, not all regulations are a form of government overreach, believe it or not, sometimes they do have your best interest in mind. Let's look at why it's important that fast food restaurants stay accountable to the people they are helping be obese. You know how every label in the world reads, "Percent Daily Values are based on a 2,000-calorie diet"? This has been the standard for a long time, and is still a fair measure for the average person. When in doubt, stay around 2,000 calories a day. A triple whopper value meal at Burger King, with large fries, and large soda clocks in at 2,100 calories, with over 100 grams of fat! More than your daily allowance of both metrics.

Ironically, as I sit here writing this, a few moments ago I took a break to clear my head. Since I am an American with my bad habits too, I decided to mindlessly scroll Instagram for a moment. It only took me a few seconds to see my first ad, sponsored conveniently, by McDonalds. It read, "The delicious, iconic Big Mac now comes in three sizes! It's like music to your ears. Get 'em while you can." Pictured is three Big Macs, in different sizes, swirling in circles with music notes rising from them. The joy of saturated fat and high calories. The Jr Mac, The Big Mac, and The Grand Mac, the holy trinity of obesity. I guess it's good that they offer a Jr Mac, well, it would be if it the Jr Mac didn't have 27 grams of fat. It might have 21 grams of protein with it, but here's a good rule of thumb for your next entrée, if it has more fat than it does protein, choose something else. The Grand Mac bloats the calories up to 860, with 52 grams of fat, 62 grams of carbs, and 41 grams of protein. There has been a long debate in the fitness and nutrition community regarding the number of grams of protein that one can absorb in a sitting, and the

general rule is about 30 grams. I could argue that this is higher for
some people, namely those who engage in heavier weight training,
but I think it's safe to say that the person who chooses to eat a Grand
Mac, is likely not the person who can justify 41 grams of protein in a
sandwich, so even if this number seemed like a nutritional reprieve
from the ungodly amount of fat in the sandwich, think again. To
round out this info like it rounds out our waistlines, the Big Mac
itself has 590 calories, 24 grams of protein, 47 grams of carbs, and
34 grams of fat. By the way, 1.5 million Big Macs are sold daily, or
550 million per year.

Inactivity and the rise of screen time.
A CNN article in 2016 reported that new studies conducted by the
Nielsen Company concluded that the average American was up to
about 10 hours and 39 minutes per day of screen time. Within this
upsurge of device proliferation, it seems that nearly everyone now
has a smart phone, a tablet, a kindle, a lap top, a desktop, a TV in
every room, DVR in case they miss a show, a PlayStation, an Xbox,
an amazon fire stick, a Netflix subscription, Hulu, amazon prime, a
Nintendo switch, a Nintendo DS, and some people even have TV's in
their fucking car! Hell, I even work in a gym and I spend most of
my day in front of my computer, and most of my day sitting at my
desk. That's right, the guy who works at the gym has a sedentary
desk job. It's interesting to see how quickly the spirit of the times
becomes the cultural norm. Can you imagine going a day, or hell,
even an hour without your smart phone? I try to spend time away
from my screens but ironically, I'm staring at my laptop as I type
this. I did make sure to keep the TV turned off while I sat down to
do this. Even though I try to spend time away from screens,
especially my iPhone, I find myself incessantly grabbing it. As if I
might miss some important notification! When I do succumb to
iPhone scrolling, I often catch myself mindlessly wandering through
unnecessary news headlines, Facebook, or old e-mails. Why?

Even kids have smart phones and tablets these days. It's a wonder
that kids ever get any homework done, and it's no wonder that kids
are now consistently fat. It wasn't that long ago that we didn't even
have smart phones! When I was in high school from 2001-2005, I

did not have a cell phone. At that time, it was rare. Very few of my friends had them, my mother had one but my father did not, and they were just coming into play as somewhat of a luxury. I began to desire one and I can recall asking my parents for one. They always made me buy my own stuff, which I appreciate, and in this case, I did. I drove down to the Verizon store, signed up for a 2-year contract and got some archaic old flip phone. Fast forward a few years and my mother was buying my younger brother a cell phone. When I said, "Hey that's not fair, you made me buy my own when I was his age," she responded by saying that he must have one so that he was able to reach her in case of emergency. In just a few years, a cell phone went from a luxury to a necessity?

I see 10-year old kids with iPhones. I have couples that come to my gym and their kids sit in the lobby, playing on tablets, with big beats headphones on and a stylus. These kids look like they are prepared to board the space ship, but they also look like they might require two seats when they get in. It used to be that nobody wanted to be the fat kid, now everybody is the fat kid. It's bad enough that kids are getting by on pop tarts and mountain dew, let alone the fact that parent's now fill the kid with adderall and put an iPad in his hand and headphones on his ears to keep him busy.

Kids These Days.

Speaking of fat kids, childhood obesity was not even tracked before 1963, partly because it didn't have to be. It first started clocking in a bit under 5%. Obesity started to slowly rise before picking up speed in recent generations, in 1980 7% of children ages 6 to 11 were obese, and by 2012 that number nearly tripled to 18%. Adolescents aged 12-19 climbed from 5% to 21% in the same period. Obesity rates have been climbing, but the kids have not. The mayo clinic labels childhood obesity as a serious medical condition, as they should. Obese children become obese adults, bringing in all the common maladies such as diabetes and hypertension, and they help bloat the medical costs like their midsections along the way. Obese parents have decades of poor eating and exercise habits, and will invariably pass this on to their soon to be obese children. Parents, if you are buying your kids soda, candy, pop tarts, fast food, chips, and a myriad of other less than undesirables, you're literally killing your kids. You are effectively buying them a life of obesity and disease that will be riddled with the ups and downs of continued, failed attempts at weight loss.

It's generally suggested that children should get 60 minutes of physical activity a day. Looking back to my own childhood, in the not so distant 1990s, physical activity was not much of a concern, and I even grew up in the time of Nintendo, Sega, VHS, and the rise of computers. I was no stranger to Mario Kart but it seemed that general pass times as a kid for me was basketball, skateboarding, jumping on the trampoline, and backyard wrestling. (Sorry mother.) It's now reported that roughly 40% of kids aged 6 to 11 reach that number, and only 8% of kids aged 12 to 19! I guess the older we get the lazier we get. Look at adults, they're supposed to be the role models!

We're clearly reaching a tipping point here. As we realize the gravity of our glutton fueled evolution we must understand that like gravity, what goes up must come down. This is where we find ourselves, in a series of which we are now learning the extremes. We've known for a while now that we are eating too much and moving too little. Our kids are getting too fat, and so are we. Our healthcare costs are rising and our energy levels are dropping. We are in a fast-moving century with slow moving bodies. In the following pages, I will outline why this is such a serious issue, what we can do about it, and what we stand to gain.

Emotional Mastery, or The Lack Of.

In a discussion with peers recently the universal question of fitness professionals came up. "What do you think is the #1 reason people struggle with managing their health?" As is evidenced by the writing of this book, I think there are myriad contributing factors. This chapter was written in the aim of constructing an understanding of the evolution of factors that have created a climate that makes it very easy to be sedentary, over-indulged, and overweight. Meanwhile, Americans have every resource imaginable to push back, yet we are heading in the wrong direction.

Food, especially sugary, fatty food serves as a pleasure center for people. Their sedentary ways of sitting at home on an iPad with the television on after work is a reprieve from the drudgery and monotony of work in the 21st century. Most Americans feel unfulfilled in their work and in their lives and these sorts of pleasure center escapes are an easy source of levity. When faced with the prospects of what we must do to reverse course we recoil back into our habit centered lives easier than we cultivate meaningful change for ourselves. It isn't so hard to lead a healthy lifestyle, but it's even easier not to.

"Nature has placed mankind under the government of two sovereign masters,
pain and pleasure... they govern us in all we do, all we say, in all we think.
Every effort we make to throw off our subjection, will serve but to
demonstrate and confirm it."
-Jeremy Bentham

It is an unfortunate discovery to conclude that perhaps humans lack the inherent emotional mastery to overcome such primal tendencies and desires, and to agree that we capitulate so easily to societal norms and influences. Man is conveniently beholden to his most undesirable proclivities more often than he pushes back against the whim of impulse and the momentum of his habit.

It is not enough to cite the circumstances in which we find ourselves as the primary driver of all ill health, but the conditions created certainly facilitate the rise of gluttony and the fall of physical activity. I believe that Bentham sums this up perfectly by stating that we are governed purely by two forces, pain, and pleasure.
 While we know that sweet treats and time in front of the TV is pleasurable, we associate exercise and disciplined eating with pain.
 Regarding exercise, it's not only the exercise itself that presents the pain. The very thought of the discipline required, the longevity, and the consistency speak strongly against our human tendencies. We

know that we must drive to a gym, several times a week, that we must pay for, to exert effort and endure pain and discomfort on a regular basis, and we must continue to do so for the rest of our life. We know that we must exert control in the face of desire, and overcome our inability to eat a balanced diet, and we must continue to do that, for the rest of our life.

Not only does that sound painful, but it is unknown to us. We know and draw comfort from our habits and tendencies, and we cling to them like life itself, even if they bring us one step closer to death's door. Through pleasure and habit, we create comfort zones for ourselves. It takes massive strength of character to overcome the governing emotions that rule our lives, this is proven by the small percentages of people who push the other direction.

I believe that change starts with education. I believe that change must come from within. It's no secret that everyone knows that they need to live a healthier life, but few want it bad enough to take long term, lasting action. I have been persuading people to take on a positive and healthy lifestyle for years, and it seems to me that for change to happen, and more importantly stick, an emotional trigger must occur. I believe that if you educate people enough on the severity and repercussions of our more gluttonous ways you start to fuel the fire. One must come to understand how truly serious of a problem this is, how much their long-term health is affected, how much their habits cost us as a society, and how their poor habits will trickle down for generations to come.

I hope to help cultivate the mindset that the status quo is unacceptable. If you come to realize this discovery you are turning your sights in the right direction. I will outline in the pages to come why I feel so strongly that the fitness of a nation has become a moral issue, in hopes that you will continue to strengthen your own resolve in the face of such ironic adversity. There is so much to be gained by the shift to a Glutton Free lifestyle that it seems almost absurd to remain complacent. We must call ourselves to action and set forward on a new, more positive path.

**"If you don't know where you're going,
any road will get you there."
-Lewis Carroll**

Chapter 2: The Fitness Of A Nation Is A Moral Issue

(The economic impact of glutton fueled obesity)

fitness

noun

the condition of being physically fit or healthy.

the quality of being suitable to fulfill a role or task.

Unintended Consequences.

Growth is central to the well-being of economies and nations, and capitalism has proven to be the best of current systems to facilitate constant, limitless growth. The growth of food production, the fast food industry, and the propagation of bad food in conjunction with the rise of inactivity has created a lot of jobs, it has helped our economy soar to unbelievable heights, and it has made some people a lot of money. When profit and growth are the primary drivers of any endeavor it can be easy to shun the unintended consequences that loom in the background as the shadow that hangs over a sunset. We see what we want to see and shade what we must. ***Obesity is the sardonic byproduct of free market fundamentalism, and a consumption driven economy and culture.***

As I sit here in early 2017, the nation is in a heated argument over the future of American Healthcare. Paul Ryan and the GOP are currently trying to enact legislation known as the American Health Care Act, and the Affordable Care Act hangs in the balance. The debate is centered on the role of government in healthcare, taxation, mandates, affordability and free choice. In no debate, by either side, is the actual health of our nation mentioned. Today I met a wonderful woman, who is looking to begin and exercise and improve her health, and she's very concerned about getting her husband on board. Her husband is 310 lbs. He has a sedentary job and he's completely inactive physically. He has high blood pressure, cholesterol, bad knees, a bad back, gets winded after short walks. Because of this he takes medicines of all kinds to calm these maladies, each of which is brought on by unhealthy lifestyle and facilitated by this capitalist, growth oriented economic model that has cultivated an environment that gives birth and maintenance to such poor health. His rising health care cost is not the result of republicans, democrats, the affordable care act, the government, the insurance companies, or the pharmaceutical companies. They are the result of the rise of gluttony and the fall of physical activity. They are a result of his habits, his choices, and his lack of conviction and willpower to take positive action.

We can now say that obesity costs this country hundreds of billions of dollars per year. It is my strong opinion, that when the lifestyle decisions of a person can affect and cost others, it becomes a moral concern. If I rear end you in your car and total it, I have costed you a lot of money, therefore it is on me to fix it. Yet if I eat like shit and plop my fat ass on the couch for hours on end, which in turn contributes to rising healthcare costs, effectively raising YOUR healthcare costs, I am not held responsible. In fact, in America, I'm encouraged to keep buying bad food. We tend to see regulations put in place when capitalism gets ahead of itself and a profitable endeavor begins to create negative consequences from health or environmental standpoint. We keep marijuana illegal but allow candy bars and sodas to be readily available in mass quantities, everywhere we go. We make sure that minors can't drink alcohol but we don't make sure that minors maintain a healthy caloric balance. Food inspectors will walk into countless food production facilities today to ensure that the food is not contaminated in anyway, but they won't say a word about the sugary, fatty food that they will stamp their approval on. We regulate things that are far less toxic than bad food for their dangerous effects, however you can probably look out the window right now and see a handful of establishments that can serve you fatty and sugary processed foods with no nutritional value.

I am of the strongest belief that obesity and our sedentary ways are one of the most pressing issues of our time, yet in our public discourse of national and international issues, it is virtually a non-existent topic. Look at the 2016 election for example. If you look at a variety of polls you will see healthcare as one of the most important issues to Americans, yet no discussion of fitness, wellness, or proper nutrition. American's tend to want solutions to their problems to come from outside of themselves, and I'm here to tell you that to fix our healthcare system means to develop change from inside of yourself. To take a part of the famous Gandhi quote, I encourage you to, "Be the change." Next to healthcare in the polls are things like, defending against terrorism, improving our economy, improving our immigration system, rebuilding our infrastructure, climate change, etc. I've even seen, "Investigating Hilary Clinton" on the list of issues most important to America. If you are currently overweight, do not exercise, and have obesity linked health conditions, and you are spending time discussing, reading about, or considering why we should investigate Hilary Clinton than you are taking control of your life, your health, and your future, then you need to re-assess your priorities.

Gluttonous and unproductive.
As I sit here writing this a few days before the Super Bowl, I saw a startling headline. **Americans set to eat 1,083,333 football fields worth of wings on Super Bowl Sunday.** Now, this came out of a Huffington Post article for 2013, so even though things are a little dated, I'd assume that this years' figure is even higher. It might seem to some that Americans are shifting to a healthier lifestyle, but the numbers show otherwise. Plated next to the gluttonous number of wings sits 325 million gallons of beer, 11 million pounds of potato chips, $2.37 million spent on soda, and Domino's Pizza alone expects to deliver 11 million slices of pizza!

I'm not trying to take away all the fun that you get to digest during Super Bowl Sunday, and I know it's OK to splurge occasionally, however America has been splurging daily, for way too long. If you think that this sort of behavior is still OK, it's reported by CNN, (and this is not fake news) that **the day after the Super Bowl costs our country $1 BILLION in lost productivity.** The article reports that roughly 16 million people call in sick to work the day after the Super Bowl. I'd imagine most of those who make it to work spend most of their day in lethargy, or on the toilet. Kraft Heinz even pitched the idea that the day after the Super Bowl should be a nationally observed holiday so that people can stay home and recover. Priorities, America. I can hardly wrap my head around the notion that I'm writing about the fact that a fucking ketchup company is encouraging Americans to stay home from work because they overindulged.

The Cost in Perspective

It is estimated that illegal immigration costs our country roughly $113 billion per year. That is just over half of what obesity costs us annually, yet illegal immigration became a hot button topic that was a cornerstone of Donald Trump's campaign. Something tells me a politician choosing to fight obesity wouldn't get such a response.   In 2014, Bloomberg reports that the global cost of terrorism clocked in around $53 billion. We're talking nationally when we talk about the obesity budget, which is four times the global cost of terrorism. Where I live, people complain a lot about welfare reform and food stamps. They say that the government needed a change because they are," sick of all the handouts." In 2016 food stamp benefits cost roughly $71 billion dollars, about one third of the cost of obesity. I understand that there are other key issues, trade deficits, annual cost of all welfare programs combined, and others that do cost more than our waistlines. My point is not to say that the cost of obesity is number one, but it costs more than issues that we list as some of the most important of our time. It's easy for us to yell at politicians to build a wall, or to cut down on welfare, or to fight terrorism, it's harder for us to yell at someone to fix the obesity crisis, because generally the person responsible, is ourselves. What was that old phrase? Ask not what you can do for your country, but what your country can do for you? I think it was the other way around, but judging by the perceptions and actions of our fellow Americans in recent decades, it's understanding why one might get confused.

During the 2016 presidential campaign between Donald Trump and Hilary Clinton, a husband and wife came into my gym to consider joining and getting started on an exercise program. Both were obese, inactive, and in very bad physical shape. The man had a bright red, "Make America Great Again" hat on. He walked in with an arrogance about him as he rudely tried to interrupt everything I said, and everything his wife said. When I asked him what he was looking to accomplish he quickly responded, "As you can see here, my wife needs to lose weight." I asked him, "What about yourself?" He responded that he was fine and knew what he was doing, and that he didn't need any help. He made sure to keep the conversation away from his problems, and any time it was brought up he quickly dismissed and illuminated the problems of others, notably his wife. I won't bore you with all the details, but this seems to be a common trend in America. We want someone to fix our problems, (a politician, maybe), we want to emphasize the problems of others, and we want to claim that we are just fine. Again, it seems that Americans now concern themselves not with what they can do for their country, but what their country can and should do for them.

If you want to Make America Great (Again)...do your part.

This is an issue of personal responsibility, and your current health status is a direct reflection of the responsibility you take for yourself. It is now time that we shift into a new era of personal ownership. Do not expect the doctor or your medicine to solve your health problems, and do not expect the politicians to make everything right in the world. If you want to improve our healthcare system, start by taking a walk, or replacing a soda with a water. We have let this obesity crisis go far enough and it is time that we understand that the health of our nation is a moral issue, whether your president wants to talk about it or not. If we continue this trend of gluttony and laziness, it won't matter how good our healthcare system is, we will eternally treat the symptoms while the cause goes unpunished. Stand up for yourself, and stand up for your country, and for the love of god, get off that couch and STAND UP! Let me present a few numbers.

In a study published in a January 2012 issue of *journal of Health Economics* it was stated that the obese person incurs medical costs of $2,741 higher than if they were not obese. On a national level, that translates into nearly $200 billion annually, or almost 21% of the national healthcare budget! Think about that for a moment. Nearly a quarter of our national healthcare costs are directly, obesity related. A study by the International Health, Racquet and Sportsclub association states that as of 2009, in the United States, health care costs make up the highest percentage of Gross Domestic Product than any other country in the world! Think that your unhealthy lifestyle doesn't affect others? Think again. If you think that universal healthcare is a bad idea because you shouldn't have to pay for others medical costs, consider that your poor lifestyle choices raise the healthcare cost in this country for EVERYONE. The researchers in this study directly back up my claim that personal wellness is a moral decision by stating that the economic cost of obesity has been long underestimated, which in turn has caused underestimation of the problem by policy makers. This study stated that healthcare costs were up to $5,530 more per year for someone who is morbidly obese than for normal people. Yes, I used the phrase normal people. We are not supposed to be obese, remember that.

In the same year, Forbes published an article citing similar statistics. Again, the annual healthcare cost directly related to obesity clocked in at over $190 billion annually, officially exceeding smoking as public enemy number one in the healthcare arena. It is ironic that we regulate things like smoking and alcohol, but commercials tell us to, "Treat ourselves" to sweet treats and deserts. You might hate the Affordable Care Act, but the ACA does a few things to help this problem. Language in the Affordable Care Act begins by empowering employers to battle obesity, allowing them to charge obese employees more in their healthcare contributions, anywhere from 30-50% more if they decline to participate in a qualified wellness/weight loss program! If you are thinking that the government needs to keep their hands off your healthcare, I'm going to call you out and say it's time to take personal responsibility for your health so that the government doesn't have to. Unfortunately, we are not at a place yet where we are collectively mature enough to be left to our own devices on this. The Affordable Care Act even funds community programs designed for weight loss, and the law also has Medicare/Medicaid incentives to get people into a primary care doctor to discuss weight loss. The article reminds us that obesity has risen 34% since 1960, and that morbid obesity is up six-fold.

Here's an admonishing statistic for you, **if the number of obese and overweight adults in the U.S. continues to grow as it has over the past three decades, nearly nine out of 10 adults will be considered overweight or obese by 2030.** This horrifying fact alone calls for a paradigm shift. As we looked at earlier, individuals are paying more out of pocket for healthcare than ever before, and so much of it could be prevented or highly mitigated by a shift in lifestyle. Employers are now burdened more than ever with skyrocketing healthcare costs, and even though insurance sometimes sticks it to those who aren't doing their part, we simply need to get America off the couch. For decades, research has shown that exercise and proper nutrition is the best defense against a myriad of health conditions, both physical and mental. Exercise and nutrition have no downside, and immeasurable upside. While it's impossible to put an exact price tag on good health, the poor health of this nation has caused immeasurable harm in the realm of decreased productivity, lost wages, and time away from work. This is not even including the harm one does to their own functionality by poor health and excess body fat, consequences range from reduced functionality to overall decreased quality of life. The same in this discovery is that maintaining a balanced exercise and nutrition program is truly not that difficult, yet only one of three adults exercise regularly, almost 40% of adults sit most of the day, and one in four adults gets virtually no physical activity at all.

On a per employee basis, the cost of obesity or lifestyle related conditions is measurable, and this cost is spread to all of us. If you are against socialized medicine or universal healthcare, this should speak to you. Healthy, active people are helping cover the cost incurred by obese people. How's that for socialism? If it's wrong to ask wealthy people to subsidize healthcare for poor people, why is it ok to ask fit people to subsidize healthcare for fat people? Among the major lifestyle related illnesses, including diabetes, heart disease, hypertension, stroke, pulmonary conditions, cancers, and mental health disorders account for more than 75% of the nation's annual health care costs. Employer sponsored healthcare plans still cover a large percentage of Americans, and when an employee is ill, the economic burden is not only realized by the individual, but the employer, and the other employees in the company as well. Based on studies that have attempted to quantify the financial burden of these illnesses, to the employer on an annual basis hypertension accounts for $392.31, heart disease $368.34, depression/sadness/mental illness $348.04, Arthritis $326.88, Diabetes $256.91, and any form of cancer clocks in around $144.01. The University of Michigan conducted a study of 28,375 employees, and determined that productivity decreased by 2.4% for EACH health-risk factor brought on by poor lifestyle choices. Physical inactivity, obesity, and stress were among the leading factors. With all this in perspective, the IHRSA has concluded, and this is staggering, that..

**If all physically inactive Americans were to start exercising regularly, we
as a nation could realize a savings of $77 BILLION in direct medical costs.**

Jim Rohn speaks of cleaning up neglect. He states that there are so many things that we could do, should do, and don't do, such as walking around the block for our good health. Could do it, should do it, don't do it. He has inspired me by saying with Rohn-like conviction, "Don't let neglect destroy your days, destroy your life, and destroy your future, go back and do what you can." There couldn't be a more fitting dialogue in regard to this obesity crisis. Studies show that eight out of ten adults acknowledge the need for exercise, yet only two out of ten exercises enough to meet the recommended physical activity guidelines. These basic guidelines aren't even that much, numerous bodies encourage only two and a half hours a week of moderate physical activity. That's less time than the average person spends watching TV in a single day! (We'll talk more about poor excuses in the next chapter) It's also recommended that people engage in strength training activities that engage the major muscles of the body at least twice per week. Don't worry, we will cover some of the basics of strength training later.

Death by Chocolate

Look, most of the leading causes of death are directly related to obesity and unhealthy lifestyle choices. I could just let that line stand alone as a chapter on its own, and should illicit a call to action in and of itself. Heart disease has long been the number one cause of death, and if you look at the ways to prevent heart disease, it's no coincidence that adequate exercise and proper nutrition are the cure. This is the same preventative medicine for diabetes, strokes, respiratory diseases, and many other. Obesity and poor health claims more lives than guns, terrorists, car accidents, murders, suicides, and the list goes on. We have restrictions for how we drive our cars, restrictions on what guns we can buy, laws against murder, and we wage war after war on terrorism, but candy bars are at every checkout counter in America. We regulate marijuana because some people still believe it's dangerous, but anyone can buy a soda and a cupcake. Obesity claims more lives than cigarettes ever could yet we regulate cigarettes and we don't do a damn thing about bad food. Of course, like we discussed earlier, American's don't want their food regulated, remember, we are big kids and we can do this on our own. Except we can't, and we've proven that. Since there won't likely be any regulations on bad food anytime in the foreseeable future, this is on us, so it's important that we recognize the severity of the issue now and start to act on this. The time for excuses is over America.

No Time for Excuses

I hope we can agree at this point that the health of our nation is truly at stake. The cost has become ridiculous, in so many measures. It's hard to consider that someone could disagree with the weight of this issue, pun intended. The current course we are on has already proven unsustainable, and if we do not enact meaningful change on a larger level the issue will continue to balloon out of proportion.

I don't want to have to call for regulation to start to curb the obesity epidemic, but unless American's prove to be more responsible that may become necessary. I recently oversaw a conversation on Facebook about a rollback of Michelle Obama's school nutrition guidelines, and some freedom loving Americans were very happy about this. One man stated that his kids were fit and active, and were never fed a government issued diet. He let us know that he was tired of the nanny state. This, "Don't Tread On Me," talking point could prove dangerous. We seem to espouse virtue to absolute freedom even if our irresponsible and reckless behavior don't warrant it. We might not want a government issued diet, but the stats are in, and we are not doing too well with our free market issued diet. If humans were inherently more responsible this argument would hold weight, but as Sir Isaac Newton said, "I can calculate the motions of heavenly bodies, but not the madness of people."

Our belief in free market fundamentalism has cost us our health, and likely won't grant us any regulations on bad food anytime soon. If reasonable regulation was proposed, our obstinate and stubborn nature would likely oppose. We are like the grumpy old man who barks when told what to do, even if it's for his better health and the wellbeing of his nation and his fellow man. I am not calling for regulation, I'm calling for action. Yet, if we continue down this immature path we may eventually need to have our food supply regulated. Idealistically I hope the day comes when we have heard the last of obesity and sedentary lives, but I know this will never be the case. The best we can hope for is a marginal course correction. Even the smallest of changes is worth pursuing, but first we must get out of our head and break free of our self-imposed limitations, and our excuses. It's time to act. The health of your country is truly on the line.

Chapter 3 - I've Killed A Lot Of Grandmas.

(Why your excuses are invalid, and how to make wellness sustainable)

excuse
verb
attempt to lessen the blame attaching to (a fault or offense); seek to defend or justify

Granny Resurrections and Three-Month Pregnancies.
Let me go ahead and qualify the title of this chapter before anyone assumes that I'm a legitimate serial granny killer. It's no secret that America is full of excuses, and that is not limited to just fitness, but in the world of health club management, one thing that employees know with great experience is the consistency of bullshit excuses. I once had a personal training client whose grandmother died three times in seven months. Either that client had a lot of grandmothers, grandma had nine lives, or she was just so used to making excuses that she forgot which ones she had already used. This same client's sister also gave birth a few times in the same time. Perhaps I'm a tragedy magnet because clients that I've called upon for fitness assessments, health club tours, personal training sessions, and group classes, have truly had a rough time.

I've seen everything from dead grandmas, to emergency medical visits, recurring illnesses, massive car repairs, car accidents, overtime at work, child illnesses, new magical hypochondrial conditions, to the biggest and most over used excuse of all time, **I don't have time.** I'm awaiting the day an alien invasion causes someone to skip a workout. There are two outcomes to situations in this universe. Results, and excuses. Period. You either act, or you don't. To quote Steven Brown in his book, "13 Fatal Errors Managers Make and How to Avoid Them.", brown states that..

"People fail in direct proportion to their willingness to accept socially acceptable reasons for failure."

One of the owners of a gym I've worked at has a son in law who is a doctor. Looking for some insight for our health club he asked the doctor what his biggest struggle was in getting people to lead a healthier lifestyle. The doctor's response is exactly what us in the fitness industry understand, he says, "I can't get them off the couch." I've long stated that the competition I have managing a gym is not the other gyms. It's the couch, and the drive through. It's the individuals mental/emotional make up and their self-imposed limitations.

I'd suggest that it is important to realize, that the underlying issue beneath all the excuses, is laziness. Recently I enrolled a young man into a health club membership, with his father's checkbook. The father was a good ol' boy, a real steak and potatoes sort of guy. He had a big beer belly and mentioned his lack of energy. When I asked him why he wasn't signing up for the health club he responded bluntly, "Buddy when I get home my couch is just too sweet. Between that and that damn youtube I don't wanna do shit!" I'll commend him for his honesty. Regardless of the reason that any individual does not maintain a Glutton Free lifestyle, we need to cut through to the underlying thought process if we want to make any meaningful change in any measurable way. Remember, this is a large problem we're facing, we can't really make excuses or wait any longer.

If there is one thing I've felt that I've been successful at, is getting through to people in a way that I can help them find sustainable ways to make a healthy lifestyle a reality. The key word in that sentence is, "Sustainable." The average gym member uses a health club seventeen times in a year. This is a real problem. When they cancel the gym membership, the number one reason, unequivocally, is insufficient usage. Let's look at few ways to cut through some of your common excuses and make a Glutton Free Lifestyle sustainable.

Common Excuse #1 - I don't have time.
My initial response is acrimonious. You're going to have to make time. Study after study on the average person's use of time makes this excuse laughable at best. If you read about successful people, you'll see that no matter how busy the CEO is, he/she still generally makes time to exercise. It's not about time, it's about understanding the importance of tasks that DESERVE time. I know you're busy, I know you work, have kids in school, have errands to run, we all do. I saw a great quote one time on the door of a personal trainer's office at a local gym, it read, "Somewhere, someone busier than you is working out right now."

If you really, really believe this excuse that you've cultivated for yourself that you cling to so dearly, do some feedback analysis on how you spend your time. Be honest with yourself. Take a day, or a week, and jot down in a notebook how you're spending your time. This isn't that hard, and will likely generate some harsh realities. How much time do you spend on Facebook? How about scrolling mindlessly through Instagram photos?   According to Business Insider in 2016, the average Snapchat user spends 25-30 minutes a day scrolling through peoples, "stories." In 2015 Business Insider reported that the average person spends 40 minutes a day liking, commenting, and probably fighting about politics or laughing at memes on facebook. The average person still spends almost three hours a day watching TV. You don't have time to exercise?

Common Excuse #2 - I can't afford a gym membership
The average American spends over two hundred dollars a month on entertainment. Someone who smokes cigarettes spends more than that on tobacco. Here's an exercise for you, go into your bank statement, add up all the times you stop for coffee, or energy drinks, or a snack. Add up all your recurring subscription services. Do you really need amazon prime, hulu, AND netflix? Most people piss away nickels and dimes daily on lattes, energy drinks, snacks, etc. Even when I look at my own bank statement for the month, I can

easily spot transactions here and there that would count as wasteful spending. A few years back when I was gathering documents to rent a house, I had to provide proof of income and a bank statement. I went to the bank and asked the teller for a statement, she asked if I wanted a bank statement or just a deposit statement. I thought that the deposit statement would be sufficient, so I told her that, and I followed with, "Yea, deposit statement would be fine, I don't need him to see, " she interrupted me with a sharp, emotionless, "what you waste on?"

She was correct. I pride myself on my money management skills, but I didn't feel the need to advertise my own financial misgivings. I challenge anyone who says they cannot afford $30 to $40 for a monthly gym membership to take a serious look at their bank statement and calculate up all the wasteful spending. David Bach trademarked the phrase, "The Latte Factor" and he has written several finance books that speak to this topic. You can even find a worksheet on his website that is very helpful to track your wasteful spending. The only variable will be to test how honest you can be to yourself. That is always the elephant in the room, as people will always shade the truth and tell you that they are not as bad as they really are. I was recently communicating with an employee at an establishment that I regular do business at, where two other employees are members of my health club. The employee I was talking to is overweight, and I've encouraged her several times to come in and join us. I brought up the topic again and she reminded me that she cannot afford it, so I reminded her that we are offering her an extremely low cost of $30 per month. I asked her plainly, "So you're telling me, that you absolutely do not have $30 per month as a full-time employee here for over a decade?" She paused, and started in with the excuses. "Well you see my mother is sick, my husband left me, my hip has issues, etc" I admit that this almost sort of irritated me. This is the sort of thing that we impose on ourselves, we tend to create these self-perpetuating negative feedback loops about ourselves that limit our potential and impede personal growth.

Personal finance seems to be on the list of things that we handle poorly, right along with our health habits. While we're talking about making meaningful change, I strongly encourage you to think of this shift into a glutton free lifestyle to include glutton free finances as well. I'm not saying you can never have fun, but take serious stock of what it is that you do with your money. I resist temptations well and my bank account can prove it, but I catch myself drooling over random new gadgets like smart watches or a new portable Nintendo. As you strengthen your discipline and learn to take emotion out of your decision making not only can you supercharge your health, but your finances as well. The bookstores and libraries are filled with books on personal finance. The skills that we learn in the gym are directly transferable to the other aspects of life, and while we'll cover that more in depth in chapter 5, the discipline and persistence learned in a fitness program are principles that should resonate so strongly and should stand alone as reasons to Go Glutton Free.

To paraphrase the adage, "If you think exercising is expensive, wait until they give you the tab for not exercising." As we have discussed up to this point, America's already gotten the tab for not exercising, and that's why I've written this book. Besides, it's good to go to a gym. Do you really need to spend another hour holed up in your house looking at Facebook? Going to an actual gym forces some extra action. You must get mentally prepared, put on some workout clothes, drive to the place, check in, put your stuff away, and get to it. You'll be surrounded by other people who are on the same pursuit as you, and even if you don't communicate with them this environment considerably more uplifting and conducive to your goals than sitting at home and doing some pushups. Home has its energy already, and you need a different energy for exercise.

Common Excuse #3 - I don't know what to do

Hire a personal trainer. Think you can't afford one? Read the last paragraph. Now, if you are living in a very low-income bracket I will cut you some slack here, but we live in the information age. It might not make you a fitness guru but you have the world's library in your pocket. Use it. You don't have to be a bodybuilder or a cross fit master to reach appropriate levels of fitness. You don't have to become muscular and spend hours on hours in the gym, you just need to get moving. If you're sedentary, any movement is progress.

Aside from the library in your pocket, rise above this objection by getting started. Go to a gym, sign up, get going. Most health clubs offer a free fitness assessment or consultation with a trainer that serves as a pivotal learning point in your journey, if you don't know what to do in the gym, take advantage of this. A personal trainer will speed up your fitness education tenfold, if they are a good. When you are considering a trainer, ask his or her credentials. Make sure that the trainer is not too deep in any one niche, (bodybuilding, powerlifting, crossfit, etc, unless you aim to be a part of one of these niches.) Make sure they are there to help you with nutrition, accountability, and that they emphasize functionality and mobility work, along with full body exercises. A good trainer will tell you why more than he or she will tell you how.

Common Excuse #4 - Too busy/Lack of Energy

Woe is me says the excuse maker. Be tougher. It's generally well known that a balanced exercise program is great for increased vitality and energy. Ever consider that your lack of energy is a result of your personal choices? There's irony here, if you're too tired to work out, it might be because you eat like shit and never workout. Energy makes time, so creating more energy will make you more efficient in every aspect of life, allowing you to get more done, and to have more TIME. See Excuse #1.

Common Excuse #5 - I don't like to exercise

Oh, you poor thing. I don't like to do laundry or clean the bathroom but that doesn't mean I don't do it. There's two parts to do this, the first is that you're just going to have to get over it and out of that mindset. If you're sedentary, and living an unhealthy, inactive life, you're going to have to change this, period. The second, is that there are so many forms of fitness these days that I'm sure you can find something you enjoy. The key is to get moving. I don't expect everyone to be a fitness guru or a weight lifting machine, but you do have to get some exercise. Do some google searches on fitness establishments in your area. Try yoga, go hiking, make a habit of riding your bike.

Common Excuse # 6 - Gyms are intimidating.

Everything that is outside of your comfort zone is intimidating until you break down the wall and find yourself standing smack dab in the middle of a new world. With familiarity comes comfort. Refer to our last excuse if you're absolutely against the gym, even making a habit of getting outside is better than no exercise. If it takes you moving around outside or doing some recreational activities to improve your fitness level enough to feel comfortable getting into a gym, do that, but don't let it take too long. We'll talk later about how you're going to need a level of strength training so inevitably, you'll probably have to end up at a gym.

Recently I was touring a female prospect through my gym and showing her what we have. We got to the inevitable discussion of the weight room to which she admitted she'd never been comfortable with, which is common. She said to me, "Well there are all these big strong guys in there who know what they're doing." Let me tell you what I told her, **they don't.** There's a strong potential that your average "bro" in the weight room thinks he does in fact know what he's doing, but as a guy who's worked in gyms for years, I can tell you, he probably needs a trainer as bad as anybody. The other truth here is that everyone is worried about their own problems. I can promise you right now that more people than you would guess, are battling their own internal struggles at the gym no matter how much you'd guess otherwise. I've been working out consistently for years but I have my battles, I'm tired, I don't feel like it, I just want to go home after a long day at work, etc. You're not alone, and you're not the outcast.

Common Excuse #6 - Your self-imposed limitations/conditions.

This is the worst of the worst. I've seen a trend in my years in the gym. It seems as if we have become such delicate creatures that we must live in constant fear of having to deal with any physical discomfort. I was dealing with a woman recently who was a bit over three hundred pounds and subsequently, had back problems, bad knees, etc. She would cite these conditions as the limiting factors that made it difficult for her to exercise. This is all too common. There's a tragic irony in the fact that these conditions are a direct result of her poor lifestyle, which now help facilitate her poor lifestyle. Talk about a vicious cycle. Poor health habits cultivate unhealthy conditions, unhealthy conditions then facilitate and reinforce bad health habits, which creates more unhealthy conditions, and on it goes.

This is self-imposed. Overcoming this excuse will be the ultimate test of your internal fortitude and determination. History is full of those incredible stories that seem to overcome even the most understood of human limitations. Don't fall prey to the endless trap of self-defeating thoughts, raise your standards and terminate your old tendencies. Tony Robbin's is quoted in his excellent book, *Awaken the Giant Within,* saying, "If you don't set a baseline standard for what you will accept in life, you'll find it easy to slip into behaviors or attitudes or a quality of lie that's far below what you deserve." I love this quote, and it's the type of quote worth writing in a place that you will see it daily. One of the things I love about it most is that it encourages you to rise to the level of life that you DESERVE.

Do you deserve to life an unhealthy life riddled with health issues and limitations? Or do you deserve to unlock your full potential and life a life of purpose and prosperity? The choice truly is yours. Change can only come from inside you, not from outside. Don't wait on the world to change for you, get out of your head and get on with your life. Decide right now that you won't accept anything less than excellence from yourself when it comes to your health. As Napoleon Hill says, "When you are truly ready for a thing, it puts in its appearance."

Stop pretending that you are so frail.
It has been a consistent observation of mine that somewhere along the line America has gotten soft, or at least believes themselves to be so. For as tough as we like to talk when it comes to others, or issues

that we think need solved, we don't seem to be so tough when the time for action comes. I've noticed frequently that people tend to cite certain physical frailties as limitations for physical activity. Often these are in fact the self-imposed limitations we just discussed. Just the other day I spoke with a woman who is overweight, in her fifties, and seriously needs to get started on an exercise program. While she did agree to get started with me, it was an uphill battle as she listed several maladies that in her mind were nearly a deal breaker. Bad knee, bad back, bad elbow, arthritis, you name it. She even attempted to argue that exercise in the past caused her years of injury, just by so much as getting on a piece of equipment. I asked her about her intention to pursue some strength training and her response was, "I'm going to need to work up to the strength machines I don't want to hurt myself." Let me say very plainly, that if you think you're going to hurt yourself by just sitting on a machine and pressing a weight forward, then this is going to be a long and tough journey for you. Quit acting like exercise is something for the physically gifted and genetically elite among us. Everyone has some sort of inherent athleticism inside of them, even if it's masked by decades of inactivity and a bulging mass of body fat over the waist.

Let's look at what humans have proven capable of, physically and athletically speaking. I'm not suggesting that every 50-year-old man who starts an exercise program has to become a world class athlete, but I'd like to prove that humans have historically proven to be capable of things once thought impossible. Records will continue to be broken as we tap into the unlimited potential of the human body. Believe me, if these things are possible, you can walk on a treadmill, lift some dumbbells overhead, and squat up and down without falling over. It's certainly within you, you just need to find it.

Usain Bolt has run 100 M in 9.58 seconds. Hicham El Guerrouj from Morocco ran a 3:43 second mile in 1999, consider that in 1954 Roger Bannister ran the first 4-minute mile, which was a feat long considered impossible, but has now been completed by many athletes. The world record long jump is 8.95 meters. That is 29.36 feet!! Randy Barnes threw a 16-pound shot put 23.12 meters, or 76 feet! In 2011, Jonas Rantanen squatted 1268 lbs. I could go on endlessly here. You don't need to be a world record holder to be physically fit and healthy, but if these people and so many others can achieve such high feats, why might one think that they should be lucky to be able to get off the couch. I will end this section with one of my favorite quotes by Michalangelo.

"The greatest danger for each of us is not that we aim too high and miss it,
but that we aim too low and reach it."

Whether you claim that your limitations are because of your hormones, your thyroid, your hip, your back, your knee, your shoulder, your genetics, your fibromyalgia, your diabetes, or some other bullshit story that you've made up as to why you can't get up and take action, you're going to have to overcome that. Do you want to know the best part about that? You can. So, stop convincing yourself that you are so weak, or frail, or believing that greatness is something meant for others. If these feats I've just described are attainable by the human body, I'm pretty sure you can meet minimum exercise recommendations.

Circle of Influence vs Circle of Concern

If you've ever read Stephen Covey's *7 Habits of Highly Effective People,* you're familiar with the Circle of Concern, and the Circle of Influence. Covey defines the Circle of Concern as a model that illustrates the time we spent thinking about the things that we cannot control. Conversely, the Circle of Influence contains those things that we can control. Often, we tend to think that our excuses, or self-imposed limitations, exist within our circle of concern, while I'd suggest that often times they fit within our circle of influence, we just tell ourselves otherwise. If we say that we can't exercise because we have a bad knee, we either have a bad knee that is outside of our circle of influence, in which case we need to find ways to work around that, or we have a bad knee due to our poor habits, which fits within our circle of influence, and we need to take steps to influence positive change.

Covey teaches us that as our circle of influence grows, our circle of concern shrinks, and vice-a-versa. It seems to be ubiquitous among individuals with poor fitness levels to live primarily within their circle of concern. It should come as no surprise, that those who are struggling in certain areas of life, have many excuses, and come up with many reasons as to why they struggle, and why they can't do better. We call that a victim mindset. I'd encourage you now to take out your journal and jot down some of the things that you've considered to be things that hold you back. Do a real analysis on each item individually. Ask yourself whether they exist within your circle of concern, or within your circle of influence. If they are truly outside of your control, consider how you might be able to work around them. After all, just because something is out of your control doesn't mean you should throw in the towel. If they are within your circle of influence, consider ways to influence them more strongly with positive action. This win/win outlook on your habits will prove to be a new source of power.

Once we take control of our mental and emotional faculties we invariably conclude that our lack of success in any area of life is directly attributed to our acceptance of levels of complacency and failure. It is when you come to this conclusion that we form a new bridge to cross, one that illuminates the power of decision and the ability to change your life. As my often-quoted Jim Rohn says, "When you change, everything can change for you." In Norman Vincent Peale's *The Power of Positive Thinking,* Peale cites a physician for saying, "The only problem that all of my clients have is their thoughts."

Just Be Honest with Yourself.
Look, somewhere along the line you just need to admit that eating healthy and sticking to an exercise program takes work, and that you hate doing it. I do report after report on gym usage, and have metrics in place that track usage per month, I track the time it takes for the average person to, "Fall off", and on average, only about 15% of members are still using the gym more than 8 times per month after 3 months. Within 2 months 40-50% of people on average are down to under 4 visits per month. This is human nature. In my

gym, we even call you, e-mail you, follow up with you, and continue to encourage you to get back in the gym. This only goes so far. I think there's some adage about leading horse to water, I can't remember. Maybe you've heard it.

Unfortunately, I do not have a magic solution for you to be able to grant yourself the conviction of purpose to get moving. The best that I or anyone can do is to reinforce the need, inspire, encourage, and let you know that you can do it. It's going to take your renewed ability to summon something deep inside of you that grants you the strength to take action. You'll likely have to change, and that starts with a decision.

Chapter 4: Time For Change
(The Power of Decision)

change
verb
make or become different.

noun
the act or instance of making or becoming different.

Stages and Phases.
Earlier I described Glutton Free as a way of thinking and a way of living. I described the move to Glutton Free as a paradigm shift. As powerfully oppressive a force as this obesity and laziness epidemic really is, I can see no greater issue to force change into a new paradigm, nor can I see a more important time to do so.

The American College of Sports Medicine utilizes the Transtheoretical Model (TTM) of Behavior Change in educating fitness professionals in the theory of behavior change. The TTM breaks down behavior change into five sections.

1. **Pre-Contemplation:** People in this category are unaware of need to change, or resistant to change. Fitness professionals are encouraged to raise awareness and education to people in this phase.
2. **Contemplation:** People in this category are aware of the need to change, open to discussion about change, but remain undecided (AKA don't seem to want to act). Fitness professionals are instructed to motivate, and encourage those in this phase. In other words, people in this phase need to cut the shit and get going.

3. **Preparation:** People in this phase have decided that it is worth making the change, they are preparing to make change, and fitness professionals are instructed to aid in planning at this stage.
4. **Action:** People in this phase are actively creating change, may need assistance problem solving, and fitness professionals are instructed to reinforce positive behaviors.
5. **Maintenance:** People in this phase continue positive behaviors, create plans to avoid relapse, and fitness instructors are instructed to continue to help reinforce and problem solve.

The National Academy of Sport's medicine supports the TTM as well, and they state that movement through these stages is cyclical, not linear, as they add a sixth phase, termination. The idea here is that we no longer see exercise and proper nutrition as maintenance, but we reach a state in where we do not even consider going back. People always ask me how I keep about my standardization of healthy meals and exercise. It's easy to me because I can't even conceive of going back to my old unhealthy ways. I feel bad enough if I eat one bad meal let alone letting myself go and undoing years of progress and hard work. The termination state is the state that we must reach, and it is described below.

6. **Termination** - The termination stage is the point where individuals have zero temptation to engage in the old behavior and exhibit 100% self-efficacy in all previously tempting situations.

It is my strong opinion that,

Everyone MUST act NOW, move to the termination phase, and REMAIN IN THAT PHASE UNTIL THE END OF TIME.

With that said, in my experience I would say that the majority of American's are hardly contemplating pre-contemplation. Contemplating fitness alone might cause some American's to sweat and burn off some excess calories. No wonder action is scarce.

Over the years in the fitness industry I've had the opportunity to interview thousands of people who are looking to get started in fitness, who are already maintaining a fitness lifestyle, and equally so have I been able to approach people who are not even considering fitness. Working in the fitness industry one thing that I've always noticed is that virtually everyone acknowledges that they need to exercise and cultivate a habit of proper nutrition. When I would go out marketing and visiting businesses, I'd effectively "cold visit" and approach anyone and everyone I saw. I'd often ask questions such as, "Where do you exercise?" or, "What do you do for exercise?" Most would respond that they don't exercise, and everyone admits that they should! Many people seem to cite their work as exercise. I've even had overweight people sitting at a desk tell me that their work is exercise. I'm going to have to break it to you, and you might not like it, but unless you are working on a farm, or engaged in vigorous manual labor...

Your job does NOT count as exercise!!

Sorry to break the news to you. Running around a retail store, filing papers, typing at your computer, or even stocking shelves just isn't going to cut it. Not when you take lunch breaks to go to Wendy's and get a fried chicken sandwich covered in mayonnaise with a side of French fries and forty ounces of sugar water. Plus, even though sometimes physical activity is a byproduct of our jobs, or working in the yard, there is still a strong need for concentrated exercise. When you're stocking shelves at the store you're not counting reps or increasing resistance, or aiming to maintain an elevated heart rate. Just because a task makes you sweat does not mean that it constitutes itself as a suitable replacement for an exercise program.

If you've worked in fitness you know that it is a truly uphill battle to persuade someone who is not pursuing positive action, to do so. For personal trainers and gym employees, we also understand that getting them to agree to act is not enough, we must get them to agree to pay money to act. While American's spend over two hundred dollars a month on entertainment, most don't want to spend thirty dollars a month on a gym membership. (Note the rise of the low-cost gym, Planet Fitness, which not only does nothing to encourage usage or educate, but gives pizza and tootsie rolls to members.)

As I've stated, the aim of this book is to hopefully educate and inspire on a deeper level, in large numbers, the imperative that is taking action and maintaining a Glutton Free Lifestyle. It is most urgent that we expedite as many people as possible through the pre-contemplation, contemplation, and preparation phases, and that we do it now. I know this is simpler than it is easy. However, I've had to be there myself. In school, I was always fit. I took weight lifting class, wrestled, ran track, even bought my own gym membership at 16 years old. After school ended I stopped being as active, stopped working out, and kept eating a steady diet of McDonalds, Mountain Dew, and Doritos. It is what we always ate at home so I thought nothing of it. Slowly but surely the weight started to come on. I could see the weight coming on but between lying to myself and neglecting to change, it kept adding up.

Then came Christmas of 2009 when I visited my family. My mother bought me a pair of jeans for Christmas, and as usual, insisted that I not only try them on, but show them to her once I put them on. I went to the bathroom to try on the jeans, which were several sizes bigger than I had traditionally worn. When I went to try them on, I couldn't button them. Even though I tried to justify to myself that I had just had Christmas dinner (plus desserts and beer), I knew the score. I was fat. I put back on the pants that I had been wearing and had been stretching out for months and shamelessly walked back out. My mother, bless her heart, abruptly and loudly asked why I wasn't wearing the jeans she bought, as she wanted to see. Embarrassed, I quietly told her they didn't fit. Later in the evening we took family pictures. I wasn't too concerned because I had on a big hooded sweatshirt that should hide this mass of body fat I had been cultivating. The next morning, Facebook notified me that my pictures were online. I clicked through in horror, as I saw a bloated, pale, red faced man who seemed to have lost all confidence. I was sick to my stomach as I experienced a whirlwind of emotion. What started as anger towards my family for posting the pictures turned into an anger at myself for letting this happen. That very day,

December 26, 2009, I went right down the road to a local fitness center, enrolled, and started exercising. While it may have taken a series of emotional events to get to this point, on that day I turned my life around and went forward in a new direction that not only changed my life physically, but mentally, emotionally, led to a career, and in turn to the writing of this book. It all started by one thing.

I made a decision.

Tony Robbins refers to decisions as Pathways to Power. Napoleon Hill cited Decisions as the mastery of procrastination. Brian Tracy considers the power of decision to be the number one tool to increase time management. I would agree that our innate ability to make a life changing decision in an instant is one of the most underutilized tools of our being. I would say that the power of decision is so strong that decision itself is the catalyst for entering and never exiting the termination phase. Napoleon Hill lists one of the thirty major causes of failure as the lack of a well-defined power of decision, with that being true, a well-defined power of decision would have to be a major factor for success. The beautiful part of decision making, is that it can change your life in an instant. Hill also cites procrastination as one of the major causes of failure, and as I mentioned earlier in this paragraph, he considers decision to be the mastery of procrastination. With the power of decision, you can start right now. (Hill also lists ill health as a major cause for failure, another indicator that you should get moving on this decision to live glutton free)

You can decide right now, in an instant, to terminate your old ways. You can decide right now, in an instant, to terminate your lack of activity and poor eating habits. You can decide right now to begin an exercise program. You can decide right now to start drinking more water, drinking less soda, eating less snacks, exercising more, and you can decide now to no longer capitulate yourself to the negative and paralyzing belief system you've cultivated for yourself. It may sound difficult, but I can tell you that not only is it not difficult, but it is immeasurably liberating. There is no greater satisfaction than the satisfaction brought on by the personal grit and determination to immediately begin doing what is right, regardless of whether you want to or not. Nobody can take from you the internal force and power that decision-making yields. As someone who can remember the emotions attached to every phase of the model as I lived them, the termination state is the state to be in.

In this state, you hold new power. The power to deflect the old ways and temptations, you effectively rise above the lesser qualities and defects of character that haunt us so pervasively. In this state, you prove that we can be stronger, better, more evolved. The self-efficacy gained through this decision is unstoppable, and the skills that you gain from existing in this state will carry you into new worlds of personal development and growth. This state creates a new level of self-discipline, a lack of which is another major cause of failure described by the man who so famously wrote about the principles of success.

Manage your time better.

As Peter Drucker said, "Time is your scarcest resource, if you can't manage it, you can manage nothing." In the 1987 book, *How to get things done,* by the National Institute of Business Management, the use of time is split into four categories. Submerged time, indulgent time, striving time, and dynamic time. The institute states that the category of time spent is determined by two factors, present satisfaction and long-term fulfillment. Submerged time is an absolute waste, and neither satisfies us in the present or does much to procure future results. Indulgent time satisfies us in the present, but does little to yield future fulfillment. Striving time offers little to no present satisfaction, but yields long term results. Dynamic time, offers present time satisfaction while yielding long term benefits. Exercise is a great example of dynamic time.

Per this definition you might say that exercise fits into the category of striving time, and I'll agree that in a certain mindset it can. Most people think of exercise as laborious and tedious, and just see exercise as means to an end. People who think of exercise this way do in fact fit exercise into the striving time category. To counter this, go and talk to someone you know who is a fitness nut. The fitness fanatic does not dread their time in the gym or on the trail, but instead sees it as a form of present time catharsis that doubles as long-term insurance for health and quality of life. There's a cheesy but fitting shirt that I've seen around that says, "I regretted that workout." Said no one ever. I would suggest that most striving time could become dynamic time with a shift of thinking. Writing this paragraph right now could easily be striving time, as I strive to finish this book to get it out to the world, but I see it as dynamic time. I enjoy the process and I look forward to what it brings in the future. I used to see my time at work as striving time, and that too has shifted as I learned to embrace the journey, and embracing the journey, turning striving time to dynamic time was not only a choice but has been one of the most fruitful choices of my adult life.

We talked earlier about the common excuse of not having enough time. I'll slightly revisit that. I mentioned earlier that the average person spends about 10 hours and 39 minutes a day in front of a screen. With the evolution of technology not only do we watch our TV's at night, but we stare mindlessly at our iPhone, our tablet, our laptop, our desktop at work, and the television set at home. Go to any public establishment and you'll notice that even while people are out and about they can't help themselves but to stop and stare at their phone. Perhaps an important Facebook notification came in...
 There's no doubt that humans are inherently poor at managing their time. If you performed any feedback analysis on yourself like I encouraged you've probably come to this conclusion. I sure as hell know I'm guilty. I woke up last Sunday, stared at my phone for a while in bed (guilty), mindlessly scrolled news sources before dragging my tired ass to the kitchen to cook some breakfast, only to lay back down and stare aimlessly at my iPhone. I did end up getting myself to the gym, and I spent some of the day reading, writing, and getting stuff done around the house, but my feedback analysis for that day showed that I ended up wasting about 6 hours.
 Imagine how far that could go? I'd suggest that you also waste several hours a day. Imagine if just a small portion of that was allocated to exercise and food prep?

Time Inconsistency.

There's a concept in psychology known as time inconsistency. This basically refers to the things that we want to do, plan to do, and don't do. It's the workout supplements that go to waste on top of your refrigerator, and the workout clothes that haven't seen their first gym time. On a larger scale, this effectively explains why the average gym member uses the gym 17 times in a year. We basically see better versions of our future selves in our heads, we can picture it, we can even start to take some action to move in that direction, but our present self is never as good as the future self that we envision. We say, "I'll do it next year," as if somehow, next year, the conditions will be more fitting, or that we will have evolved, then next year comes and we are still the same person, and we end up putting it off again. I'm guilty of this with books. I'll start with saying that I'm certain that I read many more books than the average person, as I read daily and complete about a book a week on average, but I probably buy 10 books for everyone I read that week. I have books that I may never get to, and I keep buying more. In fairness, this keeps me anchored to reading, and like anything, the more I read, the better I get at reading, and the more I get done. Yet I often laugh at myself driving away from the bookstore with 6 books knowing that I'm halfway through one at home that still has 200 pages left and I have 30 books on my shelf that I can't wait to get to.

We will never be perfect at managing our time, or being consistent with our future vision of our self, but it remains imperative that we strive toward it. I'll take the person with recently purchased gym shorts and a gym membership that goes unused over the person watching Nascar eating potato chips who won't even consider eating a salad. As Richard Feynman said, "The first principle is that you must not fool yourself, and you are the easiest person to fool."

So, the question must be, how do we become more time consistent? How do we chip away at becoming that future self that we visualize so often? I don't have the absolute answer, but I think I can share some thoughts. We've already been talking about making a decision, now we have to come up with some steps to put it into action, and to keep ourselves accountable in doing so. Regularly setting goals comes to mind. We will need to find a way to turn decisions, into goals, that yield action and create results. While it may be easier said than done, this sort of goes back to raising your standards of what you'll accept from yourself. Jim Rohn calls it cleaning up neglect. In many of his seminars you'll see him referring to this idea that neglect destroys our days, destroys our life and destroys our future. He'll bring up the things that we could do, should do, and don't do, such as walking around the block for your good health. We know we could easily do it, we know we should do it, yet we don't do it. That is time inconsistency at its finest. I suppose we would do it, but it's just easier in that moment to sit on the couch and watch re-runs of Game of Thrones. Now that we're making decisions about what we want to become in life, let's set some goals to help us get there.

S.M.A.R.T. Goals

Look, you've probably heard of this. As I mentioned, much has been written on the subject so I'll keep this short but I feel it needs to be included in the discussion. The S.M.A.R.T. principle of goal setting is old news, but remains extremely effective. It is a model of goal setting that states that our goals should be specific, measurable, attainable, realistic, and should have a time frame. I've also seen this used where the R stands for relevant, and the T is for trackable. A goal that states your intention to lose 10 lbs. in two months is better than a goal that says that you want to lose weight. A goal that says you're going to start running is insufficient, while a goal that says you'll begin by running 3 times a week and after 6 weeks you'll move up to 4 times is more measurable.

Instead of saying you'll drink more water, write down how much you're going to drink, how you're going to make it happen, follow through on it and review your progress. If you want to curb a bad habit such as soda, measure it and set some parameters, be realistic. As much as I want to tell you to throw the coke bottle out and say no more if it, I understand that we're all too human and your cravings will return. Take it one step at a time, but get on that first step right now. Don't be afraid to set your goals too high either. This could clash with the idea of realistic and attainable, but I truly believe people inherently demand and expect too little from themselves in the first place. I like that cheesy old saying, aim for the stars and you'll at least hit the moon. If you've read any Grant Cardone, I agree with him here. He is immensely over the top in his actions, his speeches, his ideas, and as a result, he gets shit done. A lot of shit. His mantra on goal setting is that he'd rather fall short of an immense goal than achieve a small one. When we really get into the mode of chasing our goals we'll likely feel that we've completed it when we've reached it, so don't set them too low.

Don't lie to yourself about the reality of your fitness level. It seems to be common place that obese people think their doctor is a whack job when he tells them a realistically healthy weight. I've talked to countless woman who have been told that they need to weigh around 130, and since they're sitting at 260 they think that he is just nuts. They ask me if I agree with the Dr, and of course I say yes. This is not because the 260-pound woman knows better, but because she identifies with the fact that she's been obese for ages, so she qualifies it by saying something silly like, "I want to keep my curves," or, "I don't want to be too skinny." Just stop it lady. You need to be healthy, and carrying around excess body fat to maintain some preservation of curves is just silly. Quit lying to yourself, your health is likely worse than you'll admit, even when you're admitting you're in bad health. The doctor isn't even forcing you to aim too high when he tells you a healthy weight, he's telling you the emotionless truth.

I hope at this point we agree that the decision to act and make positive change is imperative, regardless of where you're at in your fitness level. With this decision and change comes new power and you will soon find that the rewards of this decision will compound and treat you to new disciplines that will carry you into new successes in your life.

There is no time like the present.
It's been said before that you cannot wait for five miles of green lights to start your journey. You must act, you must get going. Too common is the mindset that waits for perfect conditions to begin

acting. I recently encountered a woman who was very interested in starting an exercise program, but had concerns about her husband joining along. He has a long list of health issues all derived directly from his poor health and obesity. He continues to insist that he is not ready to act as he believes that in the future, conditions will be more conducive to his ability to successfully begin a program. Do not fall into this trap. Often in sales we run into the people who will, "buy next week." As sales people, we know to expect this, so we anticipate it and we attempt to move on that objection ahead of time. However, fitness is not like buying a car or a new appliance for the house, especially when we are in dangerously bad health.

While it's OK to shop around for a car or a new washer, it is not OK to drag out the process of moving on your health. If your doctor told you today that you have 6 months to live unless you changed your habits, you'd change, yet our impulse to act is so much weaker when we feel like the time of actual judgment is further down the road. Every day you wait your body deteriorates more, your muscles atrophy more, your heart pumps harder to deal with your extra weight, your blood pressure remains high, and your bones, joints, tendons, and ligaments bear the extra weight. The person sitting on the couch waiting for the "right time" is being lapped by the person with a bad knee and a busy schedule who is currently sweating it out at the gym. Do not put off until next week that which should have been done years ago.

Chapter 5: The Link Between Fitness And Personal Development

(Why fitness builds more than just muscles)

"Knowing others is intelligence. Knowing yourself is true wisdom. Mastering others is strength. Mastering yourself is true power."
-Lao Tzu

New Beginnings.

When I decided to lose weight years ago, not only was my health in a bad way, but so were my tendencies. Overeating and being sedentary had some residual effects that took a toll on my work life, my social life, my energy, my discipline, and my persistence. I was tired out most of the time, I felt like hell, I had very little confidence (which kept me chronically single), I wasn't productive, and I just wasn't who I wanted to become.

I credit getting back into the gym, and putting a high priority on fitness and wellness as the catalyst to greater personal change that shifted my mindset and elevated my character to a new level. On the day that I decided to make a life change, I went right down the road to a local gym. I signed up immediately, I didn't flinch at the fact that I had a new thirty-dollar monthly payment, I got right to work. My high school weight lifting days had been a few years behind me at that point, so I wasn't really in the mindset to get into heavy weight lifting, nor did I have the confidence to lift weights, so I just got on an elliptical.

I hadn't been on a single piece of cardio equipment in years. It didn't start off too bad, but roughly five minutes in I was hurting, got my first cramp, and the sweat was pouring. I can remember wanting to get off and staring at the time on the machine as it slowly crawled up through the minutes. When I got to ten minutes I felt like it had been an hour. I was 23 years old too. This also was before I had a smart phone, and the cardio piece didn't have a television set on it to occupy my mind, my struggle to stay attentive was bad enough, let alone toughing through this dreadful exercise. After what felt like the longest thirty minutes of my life I felt justified in jumping off. I had burned nearly four hundred calories, which I felt was a great accomplishment. I could barely breath, I was drenched in sweat, full of cramps, I might as well have left my blood, sweat, and tears on that damn thing.

I had been reading up on nutrition that morning, and at that time I used to eat a lot of McDonald's. I had just learned that the sandwich I would get daily from the dollar menu had more calories in it than I burned in that thirty minutes, and it took one dollar to buy, and about three minutes to eat. The sandwich was easy, and destructive. The exercise was hard, and took persistence. This put a lot in perspective for me.

I ate very healthy that day. After years of soda, fast food, and junk food this day was probably one of the cleanest eating days of my life. The tremendous momentum from that 30 minutes of cardio exercise carried me through that day, proving that the benefits of exercise are more than just the direct results from the workout itself. That's what this chapter is about. I am a strong advocate of the principles that one gains and strengthens through physical fitness. It's my belief that the principles and habits that we acquire through regular exercise and nutrition are some of the most important concepts that we can benefit from in life. Studies repeatedly back this up, not only can we go into the myriad benefits of exercise outside of the realm of physical improvement, but study after study shows that people who exercise are generally more productive, energized, and focused, and tend to make more money in the workplace, get promoted more often, and simply maintain higher levels of discipline that cultivates success. Conversely, and unfortunately, poor and low-income people tend to exercise less, resulting in constant lethargy, mental fog, and lower productivity.

While it may be common to assume by this metric that exercise and healthy eating is a byproduct of wealth, I'd suggest that the opposite is true. It also might be assumed that poor people are generally less likely to exercise and eat healthy because they can't afford it, I'd flip that and say that perhaps they can't afford these things because they have poor habits, resulting in lower energy, less concern about nutrition, and less discipline. These proclivities in turn help create the habits that keep one poor.

Getting back into an exercise program helped me in so many ways that I would credit it with effectively changing my life. Before I was exercising I was tired, unproductive, I had little energy, no confidence, struggled with depression, anxiety, you name it. These things and more changed when I decided to change. I believe that there are direct and tangible links between fitness and personal development. Many of the principles we build through steady fitness are transferable to all aspects of life.

Exercise and Success

If you were hiring a new employee and you had two stellar candidates interview, both with the necessary skill set, both with the right experience and education, both with the right personality, and both with the same attitude, yet one was physically fit, and the other, morbidly obese. Who would you hire?

You'd hire the fit one. This isn't discriminatory, it's sensible. The properties of obesity and the properties of fitness have their own qualities, created by the habits of the individual that led them there. The fit person is likely more energetic, less likely to miss work, more likely to be able to handle the tough demands that a stressful work environment poses not only on the body, but on the mind and spirit as well. The obese person is more likely to miss work, more likely to get sick, and more likely to drag along throughout the day. The productivity level of these two is likely poles apart.

Study after study shows that successful people, however subjective that phrase might be, value exercise and make it a top priority. In *The Millionaire Mind* by Thomas J Stanley, being physically fit and having extraordinary energy showed up in the top 30 success factors among millionaires. Truly successful people understand the importance of good health, conversely, impoverished and low-income homes disproportionately struggle with obesity. Overweight and obese people generally focus on the obstacles that make better health difficult to achieve, while fit people have come to realize that no obstacle can be justified as an excuse to better health. In *Secrets of The Millionaire Mind,* T. Harv Eker states that, "Rich people focus on opportunities, poor people focus on obstacles." Our habits create our successes and failures in all walks of life, and our perceptions and belief systems cultivate the habitat for these successes and failures to exist.

I've had many overweight people tell me that it, "must be nice," to be physically fit. It is no easier for me to be physically fit and disciplined in the kitchen than anyone. This sort of negativity and resentment toward people who have achieved that which you know you should achieve, is common among unhealthy people, uncommon among fit people, and again has a direct correlation on personal income. T. Harv Eker also states that, "Rich people admire other rich and successful people. Poor people resent rich and successful people." Lastly, Eker states that, "Rich people act despite fear. Poor people let fear stop them." The same is true for exercise and personal wellness. Fit people act, or exercise, despite the incessant struggles of daily life. They rise above the lethargy brought on by the workweek, the household, the kids, or their current conundrums. Unhealthy people use the lethargy of the day as an excuse, they refer to their required time for parenting, or tending to the household, as reasons not to act and take steps for better health.

Do a google search on the link between success, or wealth, and physical fitness. You'll find story after story of CEO's who exercise at 5 or 6 am. Why is it that Barack Obama, while president of the United States, husband, and father of two daughters, managed to exercise 45 minutes in the morning before assuming presidential duties, while the mother of two working at Wal-Mart claims that between work and home, she doesn't have time? Principle centers. Principles are the character muscles that must cultivate to live glutton free and the building blocks of a healthy, positive, productive, successful existence. I am a firm believer that the principles of fitness mirror the principles of wealth and success, so in addition to the myriad physical benefits you will gain from living Glutton Free, you will experience a list of positive changes and strong principles that will aid you in all aspects of life, and this starts with discipline.

To quote T. Harv Eker one last time, "If you are willing to do only what's easy, life will be hard. But if you are willing to do what's hard, life will be easy."

Principle #1 - Discipline

In an interview with Tim Ferriss that made it into Tools of Titans, four star general Stanly McChrystals cited that, "Exercise puts discipline into the day." He also believes that even if you have a bad day, a good workout can serve as an accomplishment in the face of failure.

It can be said that discipline and concentration is the key to effectiveness. Discipline is like the foundation of a house, which without the structure will crumble. Our success and failures in life are largely predicated by our levels of discipline. Jim Rohn says that the key to getting everything you want, is discipline. He goes further to say that all disciplines affect each other, and that learning some new discipline will affect all other disciplines. As I quoted Stanley McChrystal, I'm a strong advocate of exercise for discipline. First, the very concept of continuous exercise speaks of discipline.

There are few endeavors that require the type of discipline that exercise requires. Discipline is the very principle that carries us through any time we need to do something that we know we don't want to. I agree with McChrystal as there are days that I am suffering from lethargy, which lowers my focus and subsequently my productivity, and exercise has often been a trick of mine to shake this. Even though I'm too lethargic to exercise, once I get my heart rate up and a sweat going that all changes. By beginning and sticking to an exercise program you will carve out stronger levels of discipline for yourself that will absolutely carry over into other avenues of life. If you can exercise when you're tired out and dreading it the most, you can do great things.

Principle #2 - Proactivity

Stephen Covey lists being proactive as the first of 7 habits of highly effective people. I'd suggest that the quality of being proactive is one of high demand and low supply. Too often we are reactive. Reactive is the person who goes to the doctor to get medicine for his high blood pressure, proactive is the person who's been exercising to prevent his blood pressure from ever getting out of control in the first place. Proactive is the person who has their meals prepared and portioned up. Proactive is the person who sets the alarm early to ensure he gets his exercise. Proactive is the person who decides to be more today than they were yesterday and to act on it.

Play offense so that you don't get stuck on defense. Be proactive about your health now and enjoy decades of higher productivity, more energy, and a life free of the constant maladies of obesity and poor health. The alternative is a life riddled with incessant lethargy, excuses, poor self-image, low energy, and poor quality of life. The choice is yours.

By becoming more proactive with your health, you will benefit from being more proactive in areas of your life outside of exercise. When I took on a new proactive approach to my health, I found a new work ethic in my professional life. Gone were the days of lethargic office monotony. By becoming more proactive I ushered in a new sense of self and as a byproduct gained a stronger work ethic and drive to succeed.

Principle #3 - Goal Setting

It is said that the reason we set goals is to become the person it takes to achieve them. Goal setting is a way to have more than we are by becoming more than we are. By maintaining a glutton free mindset and lifestyle, you will begin to benefit from goals and scheduling. This ability to constantly set goals, achieve them, set new goals, and to schedule new pinnacles will carry through into every aspect of your life. As do all disciplines. Start writing goals regularly, get a journal, or two or ten, and start writing daily. Write out your goals, your victories, your defeats. Rate your productivity, track your progress.

I believe in goal writing in the morning, afternoon, and night. Make goals a part of your routine, start with your fitness goals and before long you will be writing goals about every aspect of your life. By tracking goals, you will be measuring your progress, and that which gets measured, gets better.

Principle #4 - Consistency

"Excellence then, is not an act, but a habit." - Aristotle. Consistency is key to all success and is a fundamental requirement of an exercise and nutrition program. In fitness, we talk about the F.I.T.T. principle, which stands for Frequency, Intensity, Time, and Type. All four of these are necessary ingredients to a successful fitness program, but I'd say that frequency and time are the two that must be accepted first. You're going to exercise and eat healthy for a very extended period, also known as the rest of your life. Accept that now, embrace it. Champion the fact that you are terminating your old behaviors. You're going to need to eat properly every day for the rest of your life, and you're going to need to exercise frequently. Embrace it. You're inevitably going to need to do things at a higher intensity than you currently do. Don't stress yet the type of exercise, that will come with time, and frequency.

Decide now to be consistent in your positive actions, and great things will happen for you, not only inside, but outside of the gym as well.

Principle #5 - Persistence

Persistence is a prerequisite to consistency. The ability to persist when the going gets tough is one of the more attractive traits of mankind, and another that is low in supply and high in demand. Exercise teaches us persistence like no other. I can think of no other endeavor in the human arsenal more fit to equip one with the habit of persistence. That moment ten minutes into your workout, when you're tired out and cycling through every excuse in your head that you could make up to leave and go home is the moment when persistence shines above all else. It is this innate ability to summon something greater in ourselves that makes humans the most impressive creation to ever exist (that we know of.)

Principle #6 - Toughness

There is no doubt that exercise requires, and builds toughness. Your inner resolve will be tested daily as a person who exercises and shows restraint in the kitchen. I recently read somewhere this idea of, "Decide now to be tougher." Don't meditate on it, do it. I love this, and have been using it in my own life often with great success. Just the other day I was struggling to stay focused and energized at work. I scrolled through my journal and found the note where I wrote down, "Decide to be tougher," and within a minute I was more energized than I had been all day, and got more work done that afternoon than I had all morning.

There are many times in your life where your inner grit will be tested, and there are few better places to forge this principle than the gym. There will be days where you are tired, hurting, mentally sluggish, and you'll find that you do have within you the power to summon that which is best in you. This new ability to drive out the forces of lethargy and weakness will bestow upon you a power unrecognized, that will help carry you into new worlds of personal development and determination.

Principle #7 - Long Term Thinking

Another habit listed by Stephen Covey is to begin with the end in mind. While he also reminds us to put first things first, we must see the end game. When starting off on an exercise program you're going to need to be able to see down the road. Whether your goal is to lose 100 pounds, or to go from being sedentary to being able to run a 5k, you'll first have to understand that it will take time. From your current point, to the point you envision for yourself, there is much time and substance in between. Coming to terms on this early will help you embrace the journey, and as Emerson states we must find the journeys end in every step of the road. Your ability to shed the myopic lens that we so often gaze through will carry through into your career, your relationships, and all your future endeavors. A proper exercise and nutrition program speak strongly to this concept and will strengthen this habit for you.

Build those principle muscles.

Just like our muscles adapt and grow stronger through exercise so to do your principles and habits. These principles could be seen as muscles that adapt and grow stronger through use, and conversely grow weaker through disuse. Most of us have heard the phrase, "use it or lose it," and this applies to nearly every discipline in life. Just like you will build strength, muscle, endurance, and metabolism through exercise, so too will you build the principles listed above, and others along the way. Embrace this personal development that comes as an invaluable byproduct of an exercise program. You'll soon find yourself more energized, more productive, more consistent in your positive actions, more disciplined, more persistent, tougher, more proactive, and you'll learn patience and the ability to begin with the end in mind. These new skills alone are reason enough to begin an exercise program now.

Embrace Personal Development

Kaizen is a Japanese word for, "Continuous improvement." It is a term widely recognized in the business community and it is a ubiquitous part of Japanese business culture. Businesses and professionals seek constant, small improvements and developments. There is no such word in America.

It is not that Kaizen is just defined as continuous improvement, but in the Japanese business culture it is more commonly understood to be the idea of small, continuous, improvements. This is something that we should champion in ourselves, as we should aim daily to be better tomorrow than we were today. Before I found exercise, I would have never mentioned this idea of personal development, nor would I have championed it. Once I took control of my health and developed the principles listed above, I gained new momentum in my career and in my personal life as well.

Champion this idea of personal development, make a journey of it. Begin now to aim to become the best version of yourself, in all walks of life. By aiming your sights on becoming more, you will build the character and skills that you need to take leadership over all the fabrics of your life. You will gain more confidence, a better work ethic, better thought habits, better health habits, and you will gain influence and power that you did not believe you possessed.

Take Responsibility for Everything.

If Grant Cardone hadn't already used the phrase so much in his books I'd claim it first here. Don't be a little bitch. I don't claim to be some paragon of virtue or moral crusader of self-righteousness, but if there is one thing that I've trained myself to do is to take responsibility for everything in my life. Jocko Willink wrote a great book on this titled Extreme Ownership. Very few principles in life are so liberating and so rewarding. By taking extreme ownership, you get rid of your old blame list. Blaming others, or circumstances does nothing for you, aside from maybe making you look like a little bitch. When you stop blaming and start taking responsibility, you take out a new lease on life. You can see your actions and habits clearly and adjust as necessary.

As I close out this chapter, that is exactly what I encourage you to do. Before you even flip the page, decide now that you will take extreme ownership of your life. Own your health condition. Own your old excuses. Own your habits. Own your vices. Own your food choices. Own your laziness and your misgivings. Decide right now to take control of yourself, your future, and to take extreme ownership of your life.

Stop blaming. Stop complaining. Stop feeling sorry for yourself. Stop crying, stop whining, stop wishing the world was different. Take extreme ownership of your life and assume responsibility for all your circumstances, and everything will change for you.

Chapter 6: You Really Are What You Eat.
(No more lying to yourself about your eating habits)

proper
adjective
of the required type; suitable, or appropriate.

nutrition
noun
the process of providing or obtaining the food necessary for growth
and health.

Food For Thought.

In my many conversations with people regarding their health and
wellness, I have always enjoyed asking, "How is your nutrition?"
Not just because it's a great question to get people thinking, but
because of my amusement (and horror) at their responses. Few
questions prompt a better pause or silence. The awkward silence is
almost guaranteed, the exception being those lovely and honest folks
who come right out with, "It's terrible." Whether you're attempting
to make changes for your wellbeing or already making strides, the
answer to this question usually tells the whole story. I always ask
this to prospective clients, but I also love asking this to those who
are exercising regularly yet still aren't seeing the results they want.
Here are two interesting discoveries I've made.

1) Those who are looking to start a fitness program are generally
honest about their failings in nutrition. They understand that they
need to change, and are willing to listen and learn.

2) Those who are exercising regularly but not achieving the results
they want, are generally lying to themselves in some form. Or, they
will be honest about their misgivings, to a degree.

Regardless of which category you fall in, there's little questioning the need for better nutrition in this country. The downfall of healthy eating has largely been the cause for this widening of our waistlines and subsequently, the cause for this book. Whether you're trying to pretend that you didn't eat that doughnut this morning, telling yourself that the liquid calories don't count, or just justifying that fast food visit because, "one meal won't kill you." It's time to circle back to the title of this chapter, and remind you that **you are what you eat.**

A few years ago, at my gym a young and apparently fit female stopped me as I was walking through the club. She said, "I have a question. How do I get rid of this muffin top?" I responded, "What did you eat today?" "A muffin," she replied. We both sort of sat there in an awkward, humorous moment of ironic realization before I gave her some nutritional advice. She divulged some more details about the muffin as well, acknowledging that this was one of those big fat chocolate chip gas station muffins, which contains about 80% of your daily fat and sugar. Recently, I was having an engaged conversation with a woman about her nutrition. She was very overweight, had a sedentary desk job, no exercise routine, and poor, conditioned eating habits. I asked her to list to me her standard food patterns. At one point, she mentioned that midway through her day, or on the way to work, she would stop for a coffee. When I asked her what the coffee was, casually she responded, "A Venti Mocha Frappucino." This is not a coffee, this is a milk shake! I pulled up Starbucks nutrition menu on my computer and showed her what was in her seemingly harmless coffee. 520 calories, 17 grams of fat, 10 grams of saturated fat, 84 grams of carbohydrate, 80 grams of which was pure sugar!

The latter is a great example of how we create habits and mindlessly cling to them while underestimating the negative effects. This woman truly thought what she was getting was coffee, and we all know that coffee doesn't generally yield calories aside from cream and sugar. I'm not exactly sure how she thought that this sugary, whipped cream chocolate volcano of a beverage was harmless, but that is beside the point. The lack of overall nutritional education is startling, so before we can start to shift our habits we need to be educated on the basics of proper nutrition.

The Harsh Reality of Energy Balance

Energy balance, or caloric balance, is not a new idea. Most of you reading this book probably know by now that we are supposed to, "watch our calories." We know that calories are listed on everything, and while we generally don't know what calories are, or where in the hell they come from, we know that we are at least supposed to limit them. In case you missed it, here it is. Calories are effectively units of energy. The human body requires calories and nutrients, and everyone has a resting metabolic rate (RMR). Your RMR is the number of calories that you burn daily, at rest. For most people, this is in the range of 1600-2200. So, if your RMR is 2000, you require 2000 calories from food daily to meet your bodies energy requirements. The more lean muscle tissue you have, or the bigger you are, the more calories you require. The more active you are, the more calories you require. The less muscle tissue you have, the less you require, the less active you are, the less you require.

Think of calories as fuel for your car. You wouldn't overflow your gas tank, but if you did, the excess fuel would spill over onto the ground. Yet, we overfill our bodies gas tank, and the excess fuel spills over, and hangs over our belt buckles. Humans are interesting in the way that we store excess fuel as body fat. Keep in mind, the body is a survival machine and the body assumes that excess calories will be needed as stored energy, which we now have come to love and know as body fat. The topic of weight management generally stems back to caloric balance, as any time we are in a caloric surplus (eat more than we need) we add weight. Any time we are in a caloric deficit (burn more than we eat), we lose weight. The science is in, there is little disputing this. We could dig further and go into the realm of hormones and macro nutrient allocation, but for the sake of this text, we will leave it here.

The body requires 3500 calories to create 1 lb. of body fat. 3500 excess calories, that is. If you eat 500 extra calories a day, after a week you will have gained 1 lb. of body fat. Conversely, if you eat 500 less calories a day, or burn 500 extra calories from exercise a day, after one week you will have lost 1 lb. of body fat. Pretty exciting huh? Sounds easy? It would be, if we weren't human. Reverting to Chapter 1, seeing as humans are governed by pain and pleasure, even when we know that we need to replace our sugar mountain milkshake with a plain coffee, it's just so tempting in the moment and our cravings kick in, starting the habit loop that we will discuss in chapter 8.

If you are 100 lbs. overweight, assuming the 100 lbs. is all body fat for the sake of this discussion, that means that over the course of time that it took you to gain that weight, you consumed 350,000 excess calories that your body did not require. Let me repeat that. If you are 100 lbs. overweight, you have consumed 350,000 excess calories that your body did not require. That's slightly embarrassing. If this is the case, your standards in regard to what you consume has been too low for too long, and your inability to overcome the governing emotions dictated by pain and pleasure have caused you to cultivate and maintain habits that are detrimental to your health and wellbeing, reaffirming my statement that obesity is the sardonic byproduct of inactivity in a culture dominated by excessive consumption.

Raise Your Standards.

Not only are you going to have to raise your standards, but you are also going to have to detach emotionally. Food is fuel and nothing more. Only in this society do we attach such emotions to our food. This idea of comfort food needs to go. If you need a sweet treat or a piece of pie to comfort yourself, it's time to find new sources of comfort. Perhaps comfort could come from knowing that you are working to improve your health and wellbeing.

It is important to acknowledge that we will in fact need to make a decision about our nutritional habits. We considered the power of decision earlier, and this is one of the components of a healthy lifestyle that we must decide to pursue. You'll hear things such as, "Health is 70% nutrition, and 30% exercise." I even had someone ask me recently what percentage I would allocate to both. That is sort of a silly exercise, they each hold their weight, while it is likely true that nutrition is probably weighted more heavily, the point is that we need to exercise and eat a balanced diet, period.

It is unfortunate to discover that we have cultivated a culture that makes bad food not only readily available, but heavily promoted. This culture of excess consumption has given rise to a habitat that is counter to the needs of a healthy society, and since this will not be changing anytime soon. This strengthens my argument that the solution is hidden deep within each of us, and that it is imperative that we not only raise our standards, but summon that inner resolve that does in fact hide within us. While it may seem insurmountable we can break the addiction of bad food and excessive consumption.

America has a Coke addiction.

I was recently speaking to a young lady who was working hard in the gym yet struggling to lose weight, of course I went back to my nutrition question. She admitted that she had some struggles but cited that she is doing well overall. This is a common answer.
 When I got her to narrow things down a bit, she admitted that she has a Coke addiction.

This Coke addiction might be worse than the idea that is conjured up in the mind at the phrase, "Coke addiction." When we started discussing her Coke addiction, she admitted that she's still generally drinking a few a day. For most people, a few, does not mean a few cans of Coke, but a few large 16 oz. or 24 oz., sometimes even a huge fountain drink! I told her she was going to need to stop the Coke. I'll relegate to encouraging clients to slowly reduce the bad habit, but I generally like to encourage people to make the decision to stop now. When I told her to stop drinking Coke, she looked at me like I was asking her to give up her child. Here in lies the problem... **we are emotionally attached to our bad habits. We identify with them, and see the loss of them as a loss of self.**

I'll tell you the story I told her. Years ago, when I was fat and indulgent, I drank Mountain Dew excessively. Easily three or more cans in a day, or a fountain drink or two. I was emotionally attached to Mountain Dew. In retrospect, I find this extremely silly that I would be emotionally attached to a neon green carbonated drink with a stupid name. Regardless, I was hooked. It went well with a bag of Doritos. When I made the decision to change my life, the Mountain Dew went with it, and I made that decision immediately. After about four or so years of not drinking Mountain Dew, I got a craving. For days, I considered this stupid green drink and how I wanted to have a taste. My girlfriend finally told me to stop whining, to go to the gas station, and to drink a Mountain Dew and say no more of it. So, I did. I walked down to the corner gas station, bought a ninety-nine cent can of Mountain Dew. At the first sip, I couldn't understand why I used to be so addicted to this. It tasted like shit. Looking at that green can of chemical water again, I took one more sip thinking it was a fluke. Next, I poured it out and threw it away. The moral of the story, is that when you give up a bad habit, a year later, you will not miss it.   To detach emotionally from these bad habits, make the decision now, and take the first step NOW!

Purpose, not Pleasure.

Now that we're (considering) taking the emotion out of our nutrition, we can start to make some serious progress regarding how we fuel our body. It's important to consider that phrase, because food is in fact fuel for your body, nothing more, nothing less. Being enslaved by our bad nutritional habits does not change that fact, so however much we like to identify with our cravings or favorite foods, this is immutable. It's also important to consider that whatever our current weight is, we must eat to maintain that. So, if someone is 300 lbs., they eat to feed 300 lbs., where someone who is 200 lbs. eats considerably less to maintain 200 lbs. A full size pickup truck requires more fuel than a small sedan. In the case of the 300-lb. person, it seems almost foreign to consider that daily they could get by on less than they currently eat. The current eating habits of this person is the present homeostasis, which can be changed. When I was a fat kid eating junk all the time, I thought it would be some sort of departure to not have those foods in my life, which was silly, as I can't say that I've lost very much by not eating that way, except body fat of course.

I have created a strong degree of standardization in my food choices. For the most part I have a few "Go-to meals" that I stick to, and I vary it up with different vegetables or seasonings. My most common meal is some sort of chicken breast, rice, and vegetables. It's very easy to make this taste great, and this type of meal hits all the right notes. Complex carbohydrates, lean protein and vitamins. I was eating this out of one of my trusty tupperware containers recently at work, and one of the clients came through my office and said, "Chicken and rice again Steve? Isn't that boring?" If I'm looking for amusement I'll watch comedy, not go to the drive through. I cannot wrap my head around the need for food to be entertaining, or high in pleasure. Are our lives that bankrupt that we must derive pleasure from overly tasty food at the expense of our health? We live in a world that's going a thousand miles per hour and entertainment is a click away every second of the day. I'd suggest we can find better ways to have fun.

This emotional eating must be one of the biggest plagues facing us in the realm of chasing better health. This idea of comfort food has become all too common place. How comforting is it to know that your food choices are the cause of your ailments? In a hyper-consumer culture like we live in, I can see how this came to be. Just recently I heard a Taco Bell commercial on the television, advertising some new ridiculous version of a taco where the shell is literally made from fried chicken. The man and woman on the TV are commiserating about this new death taco when one of them asks laughingly, "What's the worst that could happen? You could get hooked?!" **Yes! That is absolutely the worst that could happen!** You've seen the ads before on the television, or at the drive through when horribly sweet and sugary treats are being promoted, sayings like, "You deserve it! Indulge yourself, you work hard!" I understand that fighting off cravings is easier said than it is done, but hopefully we can reach down deep enough to acknowledge the importance and the need for such a transition, and if we can decide that we want to change bad enough, we will change, because while proper nutrition is not easy, it is simple.

All you need is the basics.
I'm blown away by the lack of general nutritional knowledge that is apparently pervasive in America. I've had countless people tell me they don't know what a calorie is. I've met people who drink virtually no water. I talk to people about nutrition and half of the time they look at me like I'm teaching quantum physics. Look folks, this truly is not complex. Here it is... wait for it... are you ready?

Eat less junk.
Eat more healthy foods.
Drink more water.
Keep your portions under control.

That's it. Truly. Add a reasonable amount of physical activity to your life and you're good to go. This does not have to be difficult. I could just leave it there, but considering the general lack of education on the topic, I'll cover the basics. If you are one of the people who paid attention in health class in junior high, or have at one point in your life googled, "proper nutrition" and read for 30 seconds, you can move on, but for the rest of you, here we go.

The fundamentals of proper nutrition.
There are four things in this universe that yield calories, carbohydrate, protein, fat, and alcohol. That's it. Each of these things have very different properties and different caloric yields, but here is what you need to know.

1 Gram of Carbohydrate yields 4 calories.
1 Gram of Protein yields 4 calories.
1 Gram of Fat yields 9 calories.
1 Gram of Alcohol yields 7 calories.

Carbohydrates are made of sugar(s) and are the primary source of glucose, or energy, in the body. There are effectively simple, and complex carbohydrates. Complex carbohydrates are a prime energy source as they afford a more moderate and sustained supply of glucose to the body, and they don't cause us to spike and crash like simple sugars do. Most fitness and nutrition organizations recommend that 50 to 80 percent of our daily calories should come from carbohydrate. Don't freak out over that statement, while I'll probably recommend we stay on the lower scale of that, people have developed a fear of the carbohydrate. The only thing you should fear about carbohydrate is not burning the carbohydrate you eat by sitting on the couch while you're eating potato chips. There's a reason why athletes can drink sugary sports drinks during intense competition and have six packs, and why Joe Cool drinks a sports drink on the couch and has a beer belly.

To keep it simple - Carbohydrates have a low caloric yield, and are used for energy. Since we are eating for need, we eat appropriate amount of carbohydrates relative to our activity level. Period.

Proteins are made of amino acids and are essential for muscular growth and recovery. Protein is essential to the person who exercises, as this will be the primary catalyst for muscular growth and in turn, a stronger metabolism. There are varying schools of thought on how much protein one needs, and it is determined partly by your activity level. For the average person trying to lose weight, roughly .8 grams per pound of LEAN body mass is appropriate. Get your body fat checked at the gym that you just signed up at, and a reasonably experienced trainer should be able to help you with this.

To keep it simple - Protein has a low caloric yield, and the calories that protein generates will generally be healthy appropriate calories. If you're exercising often and looking to build muscle, up your protein a bit.

Fats have their place in our diet as well while they help pad vital organs and skeleton, help transport fat soluble vitamins, and provide energy. Saturated and Trans-fat should be highly avoided, aim for monounsaturated and polyunsaturated fats. Unless you're on a ketogenic diet, keep your fats moderately low in your diet. Lower than your carbohydrates and protein. That's it for keeping it simple.

Alcohol. What more do I need to say? I am no saint and I love a good drink, and we all should enjoy ourselves a bit, but keep a handle on it. Alcohol provides empty calories, and the yield is nearly twice that of a gram of carbohydrate or protein. If you're going to drink, consider the caloric yield. (Or just get drunk enough to not care.)

Water is essential. You should aim to drink half of your body weight in ounces, daily. This is to be drank in regular intervals. If you've heard of the gallon challenge, this is a great concept. A person takes a gallon jug, and marks time stamps on it. 10 Am, 12 PM, 1 PM, etc. These lines serve as benchmarks for where your water consumption should be at a given time. You don't have to do the gallon challenge to drink sufficient water, but it is the right idea. When you become thirsty your body is already telling you that you're somewhat dehydrated, so drink up. This is easy, no excuses. Besides, water is mostly free. It's literally the only drink or food that's free, and it happens to be the healthiest, most vital, and most neglected. Speaking of inexpensive nutrition...

Eating healthy is not expensive, eating for convenience is.
We've all heard it before. "Eating healthy is too expensive." I'll cite that age-old reference that I'll probably use forty times in this book. If you think eating healthy is expensive, wait until they give you the bill for not eating healthy. You have probably already gotten that bill, it's your medical bill. That bill also comes in the form of lost wages from sick days at work and your health insurance premium. I'm not even entirely sure where this notion that eating healthy comes from. Maybe it's because I am from the mid-west, and there is no such thing as Whole Foods out here, and the nearest Trader Joes is always a city away.

When I go to the store and buy my same standardized grocery list of chicken, lean beef, produce, complex carbohydrates, etc., I buy these things in large portions. I know that every weekend I'm going to cook up a bunch of protein, carbs, and veggies, and portion them out into containers. Buying these items in relative bulk and preparing them for the week yields me an average meal cost of about $1.50 to $3.00. Let's picture a scenario in which I did not prepare my meals.

It's noon, I'm hungry, at the office. I have no food prepared. I now need to contemplate where I'm going to go, what I'm going to get, and how I can find something affordable and healthy. I'm not going to do fast food so I guess I could go to a Panera perhaps. I can count on the meal being a solid $10, all things considered, plus I'm going to have to close my office for at least thirty minutes to account for travel time there and back, and the time waiting. So, I'm spending $10, thirty minutes, the gas to get there and back, the miles on my car, and the lost productivity by leaving the office and potentially missing an important phone call or sale. I could do this a few times daily, ruin my bank account and add the unnecessary and consistent stress of decision making, or I could walk to the break room, grab one of my meals out of the refrigerator, microwave it, and be back to my desk in a few minutes. Even if I take a few minutes away from my work to eat, I'm still present and could catch some much-needed business. I traded a $10 meal for a $2 meal, I saved 20-30 minutes, I saved gas, stress, and miles on my car. Plus, my meal was portioned at home, and much healthier than anything I could get at a restaurant.

Now just imagine if you're the person going out and getting fast food, where not only the food has gone up in price, but we know what to expect from a nutritional standpoint.

Breakfast in America.
We've all heard for generations that breakfast is the most important meal of the day, and this will remain forever true. Let's remember that the idea of breakfast is to break the fast from sleeping 6 to 8 hours, plus presumably not eating right before bed. It is in the morning that we need nutrients the most to not only break the fast but to prepare us to meet the energy demands of the day ahead. Breakfast should consist of high quality, lean protein, complex carbohydrates for sustained energy, and no lack of vitamins,

nutrients, and water. Too often now is a healthy, prepared breakfast at home foregone for a convenient and greasy trip through the drive thru. More Americans than ever now eat their meals in the car. McDonald's sells 40 billion dollars of breakfast food per year, and most of this is fatty sandwiches loaded with grease, cheese, and sausage. For god's sake, you can even buy a breakfast sandwich that has pancakes instead of the bread!

Even when we eat at home too many American's are eating cereal. Once regarded as a healthy breakfast with a complete nutritional profile, too often we go for the sugar filled types that might as well be candy that we sprinkle into milk. Between cereal, doughnuts, cinnamon rolls, pancakes, waffles, and other assorted pastries, you can see that we've got our breakfast priorities out of order. Maybe you're telling yourself right now that you'd eat a healthier breakfast but you just don't have time, and between getting the kids ready for school and rushing out the door, a honey bun or a mcgriddle is just more convenient, you're going to have to toughen up and work around it. Decide now to be tougher. Get up earlier, or prepare breakfast the night before. Remember the talk about personal responsibility? Quit making excuses.

The Power of Meal Prep.

I've already cited some of the benefits of meal prep but I'll conclude this chapter by saying that you absolutely must start doing this. Not only will your meals be healthier, they will be more accessible, convenient, and you will certainly save time. The time it takes on the weekend to prepare food for an hour or two pays dividends when it's a busy day at work. You'll find that you're less stressed because you don't have to make mundane, unnecessary decisions. You'll find that you're more satiated because your food will contain more complete nutrient profiles, and you'll become a better cook at the same time.

As we start on our exercise program and begin to accept the merits of a well-rounded program, proper nutrition will be critical for long term success, decreases in body fat, and increases in lean muscle and metabolism. By preparing your food and understanding it's function

as fuel for your body, you will set yourself up for success in the
gym. Your new food habits will facilitate your new exercise habits,
coupled with the positive habits and skills that you'll build along the
way, your character will be granted new strength.

Chapter 7: Lunks, Dad-Bods, And Soccer Moms.

(The case for strength training)

strength

noun

1. the quality or state of being strong, in particular

2. a good or beneficial quality or attribute of a person or thing.

Common Misperception

What do you think of when you hear the phrase, "weight lifting"? Do you picture a beefed-up body builder? The clanking or iron weights in a dirty, meathead filled gym? Do you picture a humongous man carrying boulders and dragging semi-trucks in a strong man competition? If you're a woman, do you picture those rare sights of a woman with shoulders so big she barely has a neck? If so, I hope to change that by the end of this chapter. With no intent to be extreme here, the myriad conversations I've had with people regarding strength training do warrant my initial questions.

Selling gym memberships, while not a prestigious task, has been how I've spent a large portion of my time in the fitness industry. It has given me a microscope into the minds of the masses when they are in stages of behavior change toward a fitness lifestyle. When someone walks into my office and asks the oh so common question, "How much is a gym membership?" I get to begin what is effectively a sales process. As any sales person knows, questions, and unlocking emotion is key in building a relationship that leverages a buying decision. In the fitness world, this also presents a fun opportunity to look inside of the person across from you, amidst a topic that is so fraught with lack of personal responsibility, willpower, unfortunate predispositions, and fear of failure. Invariably comes the time when I ask the person what they plan to do when they get into the gym, or whether they plan to do any strength training. Aside from the occasional person who has some experience in the gym, and some understanding of weight lifting, the average person has a variety of interesting answers to this.

It is evidenced by my interactions that the public, sees cardio as means to fat loss, and weight training as means to building muscle. While this is not entirely wrong, and is a fair initial assessment, we must set the record straight by shifting our thinking a bit on this. Innumerable women have responded to me by saying that they have no intention to lift weights, as they believe that lifting weights will make them "big and bulky." I have even had a 260-pound woman tell me that she fears that she would get, "big," like me if she lifted weights, even though she already weighs 60 pounds more than me. Coming from overweight or obese women this is admittedly amusing, as the smart ass inside of me wants to say, "no, those beef manhattans and fried doughnuts make you big and bulky." The other amusing component of that thought process, is that I have been lifting weights steadily and heavily for years, eating and supplementing for muscle mass, and I'm only clocking in at one hundred and ninety-five pounds, at about five feet ten inches tall. I enjoy telling the ladies to not worry, that unless they are going to eat countless steaks and chicken breasts daily, lift weights heavily for years, and indulge in large amounts of muscle building supplements, good luck. If a woman were to shoulder press dumbbells weekly and do a few sets on the leg press and end up with the mass of a world class male bodybuilder, I'd like to know her secrets.

In asking males the same question, ironically, I get a similar answer. I recently met with an obese male in his mid-fifties who was planning to lose weight, if he was planning on doing any weight lifting in the gym, his response was as follows, "I ain't trying to be no bodybuilder." No shit. I'd say he built quite a bit of body sitting on the couch watching people drastically more fit than himself rushing up and down a grass field chasing an odd shaped ball. He also likely criticized some of them vocally for their physical misgivings or athletic mistakes. I digress. I even had a male client recently tell me he would start his exercise program with cardio, in a plan to lose what he called, "the easy weight" before moving on to weight training. This puzzled both myself and my trainers.

The case for strength.
Mark Rippetoe, a world-renowned author and strength and conditioning expert, states that physical strength is the most important attribute in human life. While I don't know that I agree one hundred percent, I like the idea. Going back to the definition of strength as a good or beneficial attribute of a person or thing, I think we all agree that strength seems to be something that has only positive attributes. Based on our public discourse, it seems like strength is something that we admire. We want strong leaders. We want to be strong on national security, strong on terrorism, strong on immigration. We want a strong economy, strong infrastructure, and strong character. I would say that all those things are innately good, and that not only is a strong character infinitely important, but I believe strength in all personal facets, is a cornerstone of character. In addition to strength, we seem to be very critical of weakness. The importance of physical strength is so true, that we must take a good hard look at ourselves if we are critical of weakness in others, yet struggle to get off the couch.

In the world of fitness, strength training is often referred to as resistance training. The American College of Sports Medicine states that, "A resistance training program can affect almost every system in the body and is used in a wide variety of populations, from children preparing for youth sports to counteracting the effects of the aging process." In George W Kirkley's old book, "Weight Lifting and Weight Training", Kirkley says, "Most men cherish a desire to have a well-developed body, even if very few of them take the trouble to do anything about it, but those who do train for improved health, strength and development are wise. Wise because one of the most important things in life is good health." Strength is an important attribute of good health. Improvements in strength and musculature has wide ranging benefits, in other words, strength is all upside.

Strength has no downside.

Strength training increases metabolism. When I was a kid all that I knew about metabolism came from my mother ranting around the house that she was putting on weight, and her failing metabolism seemed to be the culprit. I didn't really know what metabolism is, (nor did she), but it seemed to be that a bad or slow metabolism was a cause for weight gain, and a good or fast metabolism seemed to be a catalyst of good body composition. This was somewhat accurate. Dr Fredrick Hatfield of the International Sports Sciences Association is credited saying, "Big muscles burn more calories than little muscles." This is effectively the basis for all fitness professionals who are instructing strength training to clients looking to lose weight. I would love to delve into the science of metabolism, but since I subscribe myself to the KISS principle, which stands for Keep It Simple, Stupid. I will in fact, keep it simple. **The more muscle you add to your body, the more calories you burn, every minute, of every day.**

Increased lean muscle mass and metabolism are not the only upsides to strength training. Adding lean muscle to your body takes excess pressure off your joints. Strength training contributes positively to bone density, aids your tendons and ligaments, and helps strengthen your body against injury. If you are overweight and have bad knees for example, this is a result of lack of muscle, lack of functional fitness, and excess body fat. By engaging in a strength program not only do we shed the excess body fat but in addition, we build necessary strength to aid the knee in its intended functions.

Many Americans have low back problems these days, which again is a result of poor posture, excess body fat, and low core strength. The best defense for a bad back is a strong core, and healthy weight.

The Treadmill Won't Cut It.
"I just want to use the treadmill." If you work in the fitness industry, you've heard this forty-eight million times. Many an eager person has made themselves ridiculous with this inadequate, under contemplated fitness plan. The trainer asks the prospective client, "Mrs. Jones, what would you like to accomplish in the gym?"

 Prospect, "I want to lose weight. I just want to walk on the treadmill."

Look, if walking alone was the key to weight management and fitness nobody would be fat. Well, let me amend that. People would still be fat because we are a lazy creation, but it sure would be easy to stay fit. How many people can you count who have achieved commendable levels of fitness from walking on a treadmill? I do however, understand the misunderstood perception of the treadmill walker. Picture the scenario, Mrs. Jones, our quintessential weight loss client walks into a health club to get a membership. She's fifty years old, overweight, and has never been into a gym. She looks around at these machines, weights, and regular gym goers who seemingly know what they are doing. She's asked what she is looking to do in the gym and bluntly reminds us that she, "Just wants to walk on the treadmill." Of course, she just wants to walk on the treadmill. How the hell is Mrs. Jones going to figure out how to use all this equipment appropriately, let alone cultivate a balanced and well-rounded fitness program. Internally, Mrs. Jones probably knows that she needs to do more than the treadmill, but to hide her lack of experience she uses this defensively to justify her stance. Mrs. Jones knows that she knows how to walk, so she feels comfortable walking on a treadmill. She contemplates that she'll one day be able to venture into the world of machines, and move onto other cardio pieces, but after walking on the treadmill for a few days and seeing no results, she begins to burn out.

Complacency sets in, one missed day at the gym turns into a week, turns into a month, and turns into a cancelled gym membership. Now she's "burned" on a gym membership, and as the old turkish saying goes, "Once you burn your lips on hot milk, you'll blow on your yogurt." Future considerations of a fitness program bring out unhealed scar tissue, and Mrs. Jones unsuccessful attempt yields future inactivity. Years later, she decides it's time again. So, she signs up at the new Planet Fitness because hey, it's only $10 a month and they are judgment free.

Uninhabitable Planet.

Planet Fitness burst on the scene in 1992 when Michael Grondahl acquired an under-performing gym. He decided to go against the grain of fitness perception and create a populist model that offered extremely low-cost gym memberships geared to serve the occasional gym goer. In and of itself, the model is great, and from a business standpoint the model is brilliant. Today, Planet Fitness serves pizza and tootsie rolls to 6 million members at over 1000 locations.

That's right folks, Planet Fitness has adopted the, "Treat yourself, you deserve it," mentality of the fast food company, signaling the official infiltration of American junk food consumption into the American fitness industry. Planet Fitness, at only $10 a month, offers huge facilities that look like treadmill factories, they have massive amounts of machines, tanning beds, hydro massage beds, and they offer Pizza Monday, Bagel Tuesday, and you can always grab a tootsie roll at the end of your workout. They offer no legitimate personal training packages, their employees are discouraged from talking about nutrition to their members, they offer very limited free weight areas, they ban certain exercises, they ban gallon water jugs and certain locations ban tank tops, and they received negative PR a couple years back for telling a woman whose abdomen was showing that she looked too fit, and that it was "intimidating," to members.

Look, I know it's possible to get fit at a Planet Fitness, and some of you reading this right now might be doing exactly that. Good for you. I'm not saying it's not possible, but I'm saying that the rise of this model is a stain on the fitness industry, and even though it helps more people get into the gym, it's possible that the rise of this sort of fitness center is more detriment than benefit. This environment absolutely facilitates and warrants the, "I'm just going to walk on the treadmill," approach that we've already de-bunked. I'd call on principled American's to not make decisions purely on your wallet, but on principle.

If you struggle with overeating, inactivity, poor body composition and lack of functional strength, is it appropriate to go to a treadmill factory that serves you pizza and tootsie rolls? You get what you pay for, America. I'd encourage all readers to find a suitable fitness facility with a comprehensive weight area, and credentialed, professional trainers. This environment will be much more conducive to your success and will aid in your maintenance of a fitness lifestyle, and your termination of poor health habits. Get a trainer that tells you not to eat pizza, not one that serves it to you.

Planet Fitness labels itself as a, "Judgment Free Zone." They have what they call a, "Lunk Alarm," and if you grunt, or make a sound with your weights, on comes the sirens. Planet Fitness describes a, "Lunk" as follows. "Lunk (lunk) n. [slang] one who grunts, drops weights or judges. *[Ricky is slamming his weights, wearing a body building tank top, and drinking out of a gallon water jug....what a lunk!]*" Sounds judgmental to me. What better way to discourage weight lifting (and in turn a proper fitness program) than by instructing your members that you will plainly judge them for these tendencies, but you won't judge them for eating pizza at the gym that they go to for weight loss.

Strength vs Cardio.

Through my experience I've seen that the general perception is such that cardio exercise burns weight and fat, and strength training builds muscle. People often tell me that they won't be doing weight training until they lose the weight, which they automatically relate to cardio. It is assumed that weight training is for the muscle heads and everyone loves to tell me how they don't want to be the guy or gal with no neck. I've been lifting and eating chicken breasts for years and my neck is just fine.

Cardiovascular activity by its very definition is exercise for the heart. We do this on steady state cardio equipment by maintaining an elevated heart rate. Cardio exercise is also good for burning calories, but there is more to the story. Strength training and cardiovascular exercise effectively utilize different types of muscle fibers. The muscle fibers used during aerobic exercise (cardio) are not too good at building muscle tissue, while the muscle fibers used during resistance training are great at building muscle. Remember, the more muscle we have, the better our metabolism and ability to burn fat. While we are lifting weights, we need to aim to keep our rest time at a minimum, generally 30-60 seconds, or a little more if we are into heavy compound movements. By doing this and maintaining an equitable intensity we keep our heart rates elevated for the duration of the session. By having this concept be a corner stone of your exercise philosophy you will be getting your cardio in while you're lifting weights, building muscle, increasing mobility, strengthening functional movement patterns, burning fat, and increasing your metabolism. Meanwhile the eager new gym goer walks on the treadmill and effectively sends his new fitness regime into an inevitable death spiral.

The other elephant in the room is the breakdown of muscle tissue during cardio vascular activity. There are two primary components of metabolism. You have anabolism, or, the building up, and you have catabolism, or the breaking down. Catabolic forces threaten to rob the body of hard earned muscle and deteriorate our new-found metabolism. Through strength training and an integrated nutritional program, we cultivate anabolic means to produce new muscle and further increase metabolism. Since muscle is being utilized during exercise, catabolism is constantly wearing down our muscles, and since cardio exercise doesn't do much to spur muscle growth, we risk excessive breakdown.

Therefore, people who do a lot of cardio, and a crash diet to lose the weight, generally add it back and then some. First, a cardio only program quickly gets psychologically stale, making it easier to relapse. Second, those who only do cardio generally strip their body of muscle instead of building it, and in turn hurt their metabolism instead of helping it. Then, those extra calories burned make us hungry, and we generally go for carbs, which in turn helps us produce body fat, without the metabolism to stop it.

While we are strength training we are building lean muscle tissue, increasing our metabolism, and maintaining an elevated heart rate. The extra muscle tissue we build serves as a storage place for glycogen, the stored form of glucose, or in layman's terms, carbs.

So, by building muscle we can effectively take on more carbohydrates, as we have excess storage space, and the demands of our metabolism and our lifestyle justify them. The protein you consume in your diet will aid in muscle growth and recovery, further recomposing your body and increasing your metabolism, your overall health, and will help you lose weight.

Lunks, Dad-Bods and Soccer Moms.

Look around your gym the next time you go in, or when you go into buy the gym membership after reading this book. Being completely objective, examine where the fittest looking people are. (By the way, don't give me this shit about body shaming. Beauty and health are separate discussions, and should be treated as such. Besides, big is not beautiful, it's unhealthy) Aside from hardcore runners and cyclists, nine times out of ten the people lifting weights are in the best shape. That goes for men and women both. The women lifting weights are not in fear of having their shoulders overcome their neck, and the guys lifting weights aren't all lunks or muscle heads.

I know that if the weight area of a health club seems like foreign, hostile territory to you, you likely cultivate that thought process through the idea that all people in the weight area know what they are doing. They don't. They're insecure too. Even the big muscled up guy wishes his body was better, or that he could stop eating half a jar of peanut butter at night, or he's sitting there wondering if his form looks impeccable enough since he knows there's a new prospective gym goer staring at him who thinks he knows what he's doing. Every expert was once a beginner, and no matter who you are you have power residing in you waiting to be unleashed.

Now look over at the cardio section. Dad bods on the elipticals and soccer moms flailing their arms in the air power walking. If you're time in the gym has always been relegated to the treadmill or the recumbent bike, it's time to cue up new habits, create new routines, and reap new rewards.

Chapter 8: Quantify To Create Habits

quantify
verb
express or measure the quantity of.

habit
verb
a settled or regular tendency or practice, especially one that is hard
to give up.

You Are The Sum Of Your Habits.

Aristotle famously said, "We are what we repeatedly do." Whether
we'd like to admit it to ourselves or not, **our current life situation is
the sum of our daily habits.** In terms of fitness, one's body
composition is a direct result of what we eat and what we do for
physical activity. Period. If you're currently internalizing
justifications about your genetics, your hormones, your medicine, or
any other excuse that you give yourself, just stop. I'm not saying
that there aren't some factors or variables that may be slightly out of
our control, but largely, as Zig Ziglar put it, we are where we are
because it's exactly where we want to be. Ron Reynolds, the Vice
President of Distributor Recognition for Advocare is quoted saying,
"our habits are the CAUSE behind everything we do and everything
we think, and the EFFECT is the circumstances we attract. For the
"effect" to change, we must change, and "we" consists of little more
than all of the habits we have developed." As the great Jim Rohn
has so famously stated,

For things to change for you, you've got to change.

Now that we've discussed the psychology of change and the power
of decision, it's time to talk about changing our habits one by one. In
the definition of a habit we see that one of the defining components
of a habit is that it is hard to give up. We are largely ruled by our

habits, many of them bad. We can be ruled by our bad habits but we can also be ruled by our good habits, and ironically, the choice is ours. If you study those who fail or succeed in any walk of life you'll quickly learn that our successes and failures are the sum total of our habits in that area. In terms of our health, it's easy to cultivate good habits, but it's even easier not to.

Cue, Routine, Reward - The Habit Loop.

Scientists tell us that so much of our daily lives is run by what is referred to as the habit loop. The habit loop consists of three things, the cue, the routine, and the reward. The cue is linked to the reward which triggers the routine, which is automatic. This explains why the guy goes straight to the refrigerator when he gets home to open the beer. He gets home from work, which is the cue. The routine is to grab the beer, pop the top, and kick back on the couch. The reward is the levity and relaxation brought on by this habit. This is why we just can't seem to fend off the craving of fast food on the way home. We create the habit of stopping off for fast food because we associate the taste with pleasure and we see that as a reward. So, we are driving home from work, it's a long day, we see the golden arches, there is our cue for our reward. The act of going through the drive through, ordering the big mac and fries, and shoveling it all down before we got home is all routine. We don't even know we are doing it, and that is the problem but also something that we can harness for good.

It's said that the routine part of the habit loop is so strong that the brain literally doesn't even have to be involved. The positive part of that is that we don't have to relearn all the little habits that are on auto pilot, like driving. Imagine if we had to learn how to drive every time we got in the car. So now it is important that we take stock of our habits and truly examine what are the bad habits that so often put us in auto pilot. Keep in mind, the problem is always the opportunity, and the beauty of the habit loops is that we are a smart enough species to leverage it and use it for positive benefit. So, when we take inventory of our bad habits, when you write each one down, consider a positive alternative that you could use to replace it.

Once you start to create new, positive habits the habit loop will take over, and those too will become routine.

Assets vs. Liabilities.

In finance, much is discussed in the way of assets and liabilities, and I encourage you now to do that regarding your health. Every positive fitness habit is an asset that improves your health, and every bad eating habit or tendency toward laziness is a liability. I encourage you right now to get out a piece of paper and make two columns. One for assets and one for liabilities. Be honest with yourself. Start with your assets first, keep it positive. Think long and hard about all the things that could go in this column so you can start to see that victories are not only possible, but you're already conquering them. Just like brushing our teeth goes in the asset column so do other little routines. Perhaps you tend to take the stairs because you know it's better than the elevator. That's an asset. Maybe you are one of the few who does drink enough water and doesn't necessarily crave soda, that's an asset. Or maybe you really enjoy fruits and vegetables, and even though the rest of your diet sucks, that's an asset.

Now consider your liabilities. Maybe it's the extra sugar you put in your coffee every morning. Maybe it's the fact that you do take the elevator when it's right next to the stairs. Maybe it's the beer that you drink too many nights a week. Whatever they are, by simply writing these down and taking stock of them you will already start to see how you can make small, and meaningful changes that will compound over time. Just like interest, habits also compound. As you start to write these down, start to also write down new assets that you could easily start adding to your asset column, and start on at least one right away. Once you start to create one new positive habit you'll find that it's even easier to start the next, and the next, and momentum will begin to carry you to better health. Look for double positives while you're at it, here's an example.

A pack of cigarettes here in Indiana averages about $6 a pack after taxes, which is one of the lowest in the country, and apparently set to raise soon. Let's say you smoke a pack a day. You know this is bad for you and is probably one of the worst health habits in modern history. So, not only is it killing your respiratory system, it's also killing your bank account. If we average a pack a day, and the average month has 30 days, we are looking at $180 per month. Looking at it annually, to smoke 365 packs a year costs $2,190. Over the course of the next 5 years, not even considering inflation or tax increases on cigarettes, you will have spent $10,950. So not only are we down $10,950, let's look at how that money could go to work for us.

Instead of smoking, let's put that $2,190 in a low-cost index fund that tracks the market. For the greater part of 70 years the market generally returns right around 10% annually. So, we put that $2,190 in the market, and that first year it gains 10%. Then we put another $2,190, and another 10%, and we do that for the five years that we were going to be smoking. At the end of the 5 years through the power of compound interest we turned the $10,950 that we were going to spend on cigarettes into $14,707 that is now in a constantly growing index fund. Six minutes is considered the average time it takes to smoke a cigarette, so for the person who smokes 20 a day that is 2 hours out of their day spent smoking cigarettes. Some of that is spent while driving but a lot of that is just time taken out of the day. In one year that is not only $2,190 spent, but 730 hours invested in smoking cigarettes. That's over 30 days. One month, or one 12th of your year is spent smoking cigarettes. Over the course of 5 years that is 3,650 hours.

So, you have two choices. In your liabilities column is your horrible smoking habit that kills your health and costs your $10,950 in 5 years and 3,650 hours of your life. Or, you have in the asset column $14,707 in an index fund, an extra 3,650 hours of your life (which is fleeting, in case you forgot), and better lungs and health to go along with it. This ends up being a triple positive. More money, more time, better health. The only resource scarcer than money is time, and I wouldn't spend copious amounts of both destroying your health. The choice is yours.

Start First With Small Disciplines.

There's a great saying out there that states, "Successful people do all the small things that unsuccessful people don't do." I believe that having discipline with the smallest of habits is the foundation for all good things to happen. My often-quoted Jim Rohn was credited with saying, "We all pity the man who wants to stride out of his house and straighten out the corporation, has not yet straightened out his garage." There is much to be drawn from this quote, and much to be gained. They say that if you'll be faithful when the amounts are small, they'll make you a ruler, when the amounts are many. Do not neglect the smallest of disciplines.

Success in a shift to lifelong wellness starts with an apple a day. It starts with not skipping breakfast. It starts with the walk around the block you neglect no longer. It starts with using the gym membership you've been paying for that has been unused. Possibility starts with the smallest of changes. Do not neglect the smallest of things you can change for your better health. All things compound, so that 12 oz. soda you replace with a water might only save you 40 grams of sugar today, but after a week you've consumed 280 less grams of sugar. After 365 days, you've consumed 14,600 less grams of sugar. Let's say you're a heavy soda drinker who drinks 2 a day. One year after making the small change of replacing your soda with water yields you a sugar savings of 29,200 grams. 29,200 grams of sugar equates to 116,800 calories. Since we know that it takes 3,500 calories to create a pound of fat, that soda accounted for 33.4 lbs. of fat that year! Let's also look at the money you've saved. At the grocery store I go to, a 12 pack of coke is generally $4.99, or 42 cents per can. So, by switching out to water and refilling our bottle, we save $303 a year. By making the change from 2 sodas a day to water, in one years' time you will have saved $303 and lost 33.4 lbs. Not a bad deal.

Disciplined habits create more time, more freedom, more accomplishments, and better quality of life. The smallest of habits become building blocks for larger change, which just like interest compound and thicken over time. Look at someone you know who just can't seem to get it together, be it in the realm of work, health, relationships, anything. An analysis of their habit will show invariably some disarray on a very basic level. The guy who can't get up in the morning, who can't plan his meals the night before, who forgets to pay his bill on time, who leaves dishes in the kitchen sink, likely isn't the guy heading the new research program at the company or moving up the corporate ladder. Climb the ladder one rung at a time. Don't miss the easy shots if you want the ball in your hands when the game is on the line.

Minimum Exercise Recommendations

The American College of Sports Medicine (ACSM) has established minimum guidelines for cardiovascular, or cardiorespiratory exercise, resistance exercise, flexibility exercise, and neuromotor exercise. These recommendations are widely recognized by the fitness community so they will be used here.

Regarding cardiovascular exercise, it is recommended that adults get at least 150 minutes of moderate-intensity exercise per week. This is simple enough to break down into 5 bouts of 30 minutes, or any variation. Exercise intensity is generally subjective to the self so if you're foregoing a personal trainer, try to be honest with yourself. You're never cheating anyone but yourself. Consider that cardio exercise is not limited to our perceptions of "cardio" equipment in the gym. Cardiovascular exercise is any exercise that tasks the cardiovascular system, or to put it simply, maintains an elevated heart rate. This can be achieved through focused strength training as well. A good tip for you to incorporate cardiovascular exercise while you are strength training is to keep your rest time low, about 30-60 seconds between sets. Don't be "that guy" who does a set of weights and then sits on his phone for 5 minutes scrolling through instagram pictures of people who are in better shape than himself. The ACSM says that one continuous session or multiple short exercise sessions throughout the day will suffice if it amounts to the same, but I would suggest that you aim for one focused exercise session, particularly at a gym, aside from exercise such as outdoor biking or running. A gym session will grant greater results, likely. I've always told clients that one of the most important obstacles they must overcome, is simply walking in the gym. Once you're in, you're good to go. You're going to do something. You're not going to walk in, pretend like you forgot something and leave. At least I hope not, and if you've made it this far through this book I'd assume you're not that person. At the gym, you'll benefit from a variety of equipment and an atmosphere that facilitates and encourages positive action.

When it comes to resistance training, also known as strength training, or more widely looked at as weight training, it's recommended that adults should train each major muscle group two to three days each week. Two to four sets per exercise is generally appropriate, and for your reference, it's understood that higher repetition ranges (12-20) are appropriate for muscular endurance, moderate repetition ranges (8-12) are appropriate for overall muscular development, and lower rep ranges at higher weight (3-5) are appropriate for strength and power. Some fitness trainers will disagree on the distinctions between rep ranges, but for most folks this is a fair rule of thumb. Remember, we adapt to what we do. With this said, progressive resistance, or progressive overload is a must. If I grab a twenty-pound dumbbell and press it above my head 10 times, and I do this often, my muscles will adapt to that and I will become very good at that. However, if I don't move up in weight, or reps, or vary my exercise, I will hit a plateau.

For flexibility exercise, it's recommended that adults should perform flexibility exercises at least two to three days of week to increase range of motion. Stretches should generally be held for 10-30 seconds, to the point of moderate discomfort or tightness. Repeat each stretch two to four times, to accumulate about 60 seconds per stretch. I'm a big advocate of fitness for mobility, which is a close relative to flexibility, as I've noted there are a large percentage of folks who are so tight and inflexible that they can barely bend at the hips! Getting in and out of a chair should not be a struggle.

Lastly, we look at neuromotor exercise. This probably sounds confusing already, but it is not. Neuromotor exercise is more commonly known as functional fitness training. It's recommended that exercises involving motor skills such as balance, agility, and coordination should be performed 20-30 minutes per day. Keep in mind that often you can blend resistance training, cardiovascular exercise, neuromotor training, and flexibility training into one training session. Functional fitness is in high demand these days. Functional fitness is the bridge to proper movement, it's needed because unfortunately we are so overweight and out of shape that many of us struggle to bend down to tie our shoes, to pick something up over head, to squat down to grab something, or to bend over to deadlift a weight from the ground. There should be strong emphasis on functionality in your training. If you're confused, hire a credentialed personal trainer.

Force the Habit.
Now that we've talked about the habit loop, the difference in habit assets and liabilities, starting with small disciplines, and outlined what sort of exercise requirements you need to be completing, we need to start forcing positive habits. Remember the routine part of the habit loop, this can be your greatest ally if you start forcing habits. Write down now some measurable habits you want to start this week. It could be exercising 3 times a week. It could be cutting fast food from 3 visits down to 2, then to 1, then to 0. It might not necessarily be easy, but if you make a game plan, journal it, and refer to it often, you will begin to see measurable change. The hardest part is having the willpower, so you're going to have to force it. Remember, don't be a little bitch. Your health is on the line.

You don't want to grab a water today instead of a soda? You're going to have to force it. You don't want to go out and exercise today? You're going to have to force it. By doing just that not only will you set in motion the inertia that will make this habit a building block of your life, but it will help you develop that discipline muscle and that decision muscle as well. Eventually your habit loop will take over and you'll start to see that your liabilities column will shrink, and your asset column will grow.

Track now, Instinct Later.
We've all heard a litany of phrases regarding habits and the time it takes to form one. I think the common time frame is something like

24 days, but we've all heard different numbers, and nothing is absolute. There's no magic time frame to create habits, and we're all different. However, what we do need to do is to try to create habits through quantifiable means. It means that we must commit to a bit of work, but by doing so we can get to a point where positive habits are created and our health is on auto pilot. When I started eating healthier and losing weight, I can remember pacing the grocery store for hours reading label after label to get a feel for what I was really putting in my body. The first revelation was that the food available in America, or at least the food that we tend to gravitate to for convenience, is so pervasively unhealthy that one could think it's a conspiracy to keep us fat. Through these grocery store audits, I came to the realization that I pretty much needed to turn my eating habits around 100%. I set up basic standards for myself, and I set up some basic nutritional standards that would rule out most food. For example, if I grabbed something and the fat was higher than the protein, I put it back. If the carbohydrates were more than say 25% sugar, no chance.

You don't have to scale the grocery stores or read every label, but you do need to start tracking some things. As I've already asked you to write some stuff down in this chapter, you should be keeping a journal. Start creating a habit and goals journal. Get myfitnesspal on your phone and start logging your food. The habit loop is so strong that eventually you won't need to track what you once had to track so diligently. Start now. Tomorrow at the latest. Take tonight to think it over.

Chapter 9: A Paradigm Shift

paradigm

noun

a typical example or pattern of something; a model

A Course Correction.

If you're still with me up to this point I hope that you agree that the status quo is no longer acceptable. This current paradigm almost seems an ironic twist of fate, or some cosmic joke, that the evolution of our species and subsequently our technologies, that we have moved from scarcity to surplus, without considering the implications or byproducts of the latter. This amelioration of rations is inherently positive, but it seems that while the faculties that we've created to aid in the survival and propagation of life have outran the evolution of our more primal tendencies. It is no secret that the human condition is a fallible thing, and that we must now raise the standards that we hold ourselves to. If you look at human history you'll see a litany of things that we've created for the greater good that have caused unintended harm. It seems to be a trick of nature to tempt us with our own creations. In the aim of efficiency and productivity we have learned to produce massive amounts of food at unbelievably low costs. We could feed the world. Yet here we are in America, housing 5% of the world's population, while consuming roughly 25% of the world's resources, and while two thirds of us are now overweight, there are folks in other countries who don't have clean water today or a few square meals. The bible equates gluttons with drunkards, and Ralph Emerson says, "Men live in their fancy, like drunkards whose hands are too soft and tremulous for successful labor."

It seems as if the cranes of evolution that we've created such as agriculture, industry, and technology, while being the greatest tangible and extraordinary extensions of the human mind, have grown at a rate that has outrun the growth of our character. Our most undesirable proclivities shine through with so much at our disposal. This current paradigm must come to an end. We must re-paint the map. As a culture, and as a people we are going to have to begin to push back against the excesses brought on by industry and commerce, and learn to do what is right, when it is needed, whether we like to or not. Every person who decides to move forward in their life Glutton Free, is a beacon of hope that radiates to those around him or her. Quoting Ralph Waldo Emerson again I will write, "Your actions shout so loudly in my ears that I cannot hear what you say."

Resonance and Adaptation.

When you go Glutton Free, this will resonate, others will see this. There will always be resistance, but we must win the war one step a time. Reduce your glutton footprint, be part of a better way, and help us move forward in a new direction. Henry David Thoreau is quoted saying, "I know of no more encouraging fact than the unquestionable ability of man to elevate his life by conscious endeavor." I hope that in this book you have found some power within yourself to be the change that I know you want to be. Nobody likes being tired all the time, or riddled with illnesses, and presumably, nobody likes being overweight. If you are out of shape and used to the way you are feeling, let me tell you that is not the way it has to be! What story do you want to write for yourself? Do you want to be among the masses who let the spirit of the times drag you down with it? Do you want to be another number on the obesity charts? Or do you want to be among the company of winners, among those who have surpassed expectations, broke societal norms, and among those who have proven that our self-imposed limitations are not inescapable? You have residing within you right now, the power to change anything about yourself that you want to, no matter how big. Do you want to lose 100 lbs.? You can do it. Do you want to be able to run 5 miles? You can do it. Do you simply want to have energy to get through the day without feeling the nag of constant lethargy? You can do it.

In my time as a fitness trainer I've had myriad clients tell me that they cannot do something. I always remind them that my training prescriptions are not arbitrary, and that I wouldn't ask them to do it, if I wasn't certain they could do it, and invariably they do it, with much more ease than expected. I love the look on the face of someone who handled something with relative ease, that moments prior they believed to be impossible. It is an irrefutable law of nature that we limit our potential with our belief systems, and breaking through these belief systems can be one of the most liberating and empowering abilities of the human mind and body.

With work comes experience and self-efficacy, and with self-efficacy comes confidence, and with confidence comes internal power and passage into new worlds. A man walked into my office recently who after months of paying for a gym membership, decided to come in a month ago to see if he could get back in the swing of things. We had a great chat and I aimed to empower him to re-start and make it stick. A month later he's been coming in daily, and in just a month's time he's showing measurable progress. He feels better, he's getting stronger, he's losing weight, and as he told me the other day, he went from feeling awkward and in the way in the weight room, to feeling like he's one of the veterans here. Stepping out of our comfort zones is how we create new comfort zones. It is easy to stay at home and sit on the couch, and just do what you're comfortable with. You're used to your habits and the places you occupy, the place you've worked at for ten years was the most frightening and uncomfortable setting in the world the first day you walked in, now you can stroll in late with the casual nonchalance of someone who has self-efficacy, confidence, and experience.

It is the backbone of evolution that we adapt to what we do. "There is nothing that training cannot do," says Mark Twain, "Nothing is above its reach. It can turn bad morals to good, it can destroy bad principles and recreate good ones, it can lift men to angelship." In fitness, we call it the "SAID Principle." SAID stands for, "Specific Adaptations to Imposed Demands." This answers questions in life far wider ranging than fitness. If you want to get better at managing your money, study personal finance. If you want to learn how to cook, practice cooking and study. If you want to be a better reader, practice reading. If you want to be better at making decisions, practice making strong decisions. If you want to be better at time management, study and start working on managing your time. If you want to improve your bench press, bench more, if you want to be a better runner, run more. If you want to go Glutton Free and terminate your old behaviors, start changing your habits now and they will become reality for years to come. If you sit on the couch eating potato chips every night, well, you will become very efficient in that task and your body will form the shape of those habits as well. Perhaps it already has.

As you go forward now in a new direction I encourage you to begin with the end in mind, but to see the journey's end in every step of the road along the way. Enjoy the process, as they say, but don't lose sight of the end game. We often speak of adopting a healthier lifestyle, but too often our whims and tendencies of transience play us false, and our new diet plan or exercise routine fizzles out after days, weeks, or months, just to find us back where we started. To steal a phrase from Benjamin Graham's *The Intelligent Investor*, this is the difference between investment, and speculation. I've often found that economics presents a numerical measurement of our tendencies, and often the strategies, fluctuations, and long-term patterns of the stock market are a fair analogy for most human endeavors.

Investment vs speculation

Investment vs speculation is like a healthy lifestyle vs fad diets. The true value and results to be expected by the fitness lifestyle are found most meritoriously in a "buy and hold" approach to lifelong wellness. Just as the speculative investor seeks to find a way around the true path of emotionless, long term investing, so does the fad dieter who seeks quick results. He gambles and bets on hope, in search of a quick fix, seeking a diet pill or a fad program. The intelligent investor invests in stocks in which the day to day fluctuations in value or share price are inconsequential, as he who invests intelligently in paths of sustainable methods of wellness need not concern himself with the daily fluctuations of whim, impulse of habit or vice. He knows that by investing in a lifestyle of lifelong wellness, his results will compound, and the dividends of better health will continue to reinvest themselves.

Human nature mimics itself in all avenues. Our habits with health rhyme with our habits on all other aspects of life, as our habits are shaped by our character, and our character is inescapable. Emerson reminds us that all the sallies of our will are rounded in by the whole of our being, just as the peaks of the mountains are rounded out by the curve of the sphere when looked at from afar. The fallibility of the human condition is a byproduct of our emotions that prove to be a constant in this sea of variables that we call life. Be like the intelligent investor. Invest yourself now in a new paradigm, a paradigm of principle and strength. The emotionless, long term approach to wellness has a rigidity proven stalwart through peaks and valleys alike, as time proves its merits unmatched against the tide of fluctuations of life, and of whim. Up close, the peaks and valleys of our day to day life are magnified, but if you zoom out, and see the bigger picture, all that matters is that you are heading in the right direction. The two parts to success in an endeavor are doing the right things, and time. If you are doing the right things, over time, you will trend in the right direction.

Power of Inertia.

Inertia is defined as a tendency to do nothing, or remain unchanged. To overcome an object's inertia, force must be applied. The force to change must be stronger than the force of our current path, and sometimes, this requires something drastic. Let me cite a passage from John C. Maxwell's *Attitude 101.*

"While hopping along one day, a frog happened to slip into a very large pothole along a country road. All of his attempts at jumping out were in vain. Soon a rabbit came upon the frog trapped in the hole and offered to help him out. He, too, failed. After various animals from the forest made three or four gallant attempts to help the poor frog out, they finally gave up. "We'll go back and get you some food," they said. "It looks like you're going to be here for a while." However, not long after they took

off to get food, they heard the frog hopping along after them. They couldn't believe it! "We thought you couldn't get out!" They exclaimed. "Oh, I couldn't," replied the frog. "But you see, there was a big truck coming right at me, and I had to."

Too often we remain stubborn and obstinate in our current paradigm of habits and activities. Many people don't look at hiring a personal trainer, or beginning to eat right, until they have gone so far in the wrong direction that change, while still seeming insurmountable, becomes necessary. Too often we are the frog who can't find a way out of our current situation until the truck comes head on, proving to us that we had inside the ability for change all along. This is the guy who finally shows up at the gym when the doctor tells him that he is going to die. I have seen countless prospects whom looking a list of their maladies, don't find the inner will to change even when the list is a page long. Be the frog who knows that the truck will come inevitably, be proactive, and start getting out of the hole now. Don't wait until the last minute to get started.

As Mark Twain said, "The key to getting ahead is getting started." Lao Tzu is quoted saying, "The journey of a thousand miles starts with a single step." I've long told my gym goers that the hardest part of the workout is getting in the front door. For most people, the hardest thing is getting off the couch. Newton taught us what we need to know about objects in rest and objects in motion. Inertia proves itself obstinate for those at rest, and uses momentum in its favor for those in motion.

Objects on the couch tend to stay on the couch, and they get pretty good at it while they are at it. You must now take the first step to overcome your resting inertia, which will prove as stubborn as your bad habits. You're going to have to push, and you're probably going to have to push again, but just like a heavy stone that seems so hard to move at first, once you get rolling you will be unstoppable.
 Consider this book, and the power of my conviction as the hands that help you push that stone over the first bump.

Mind Over Matter.

There has been much written in recent years about the power of the mind, and the Law of Attraction. If you're unfamiliar with the Law of Attraction, the basic premise is that what you think about is what the universe creates for you. This is the idea behind those successful people who have focused persistently about their successes, and those struggling folks who can't help but think about and identify with their struggles and anticipated future problems. This is all true, but I think it's important to have a dialogue on this. A few years ago, someone asked me if I believed in the Law of Attraction, I said yes, and they proceeded to ask me, "So, you think that if you think about something, it becomes true?" Of course not. If that were true, this book would already be a best seller and America would be the healthiest nation on earth. What I do believe however, is that everything starts with thought. It must start with thought. Jim Rohn likened the mind to a mental factory, and stated that everything you absorb are like the ingredients of this mental factory, so it's very important that you be careful what you think about.

This whole idea that everything starts with thought is the basic premise of this book. I was recently talking to someone about the book I was writing, and they reminded me that I wasn't writing about a very popular topic, and I did not disagree. With that said, the origins of this book came from my belief that the paradigm shift of the nation to a healthier state was something that had to begin with thought. Very little, overall, is discussed in the national discourse on the topic of health and its relationship to personal responsibility. I thought to myself, however idealistic, that if I can strike a chord in the hearts and minds of the readers, however so few they may be, that I can start something positive that creates momentum in the right direction. It is my hopes that I have done that, if even ever so slightly. Every person that I touch in a positive way, who takes a new direction on their health, is a victory of proportions I could have never reached had I not sat down and put pencil to paper. This is too serious a topic to ignore, and ignored it has been for decades. I know that the task that lies ahead is not to be taken lightly. I know that inertia and momentum are currently against us, but as every evil that has been overturned in the past, so can this. If we truly believe in the promise of this human experiment than this is something that we must do.

Call to Action.

As you close this book I ask you to reflect. Reflect upon what we've covered. I'm asking you to reflect upon this rise of gluttony that we have enabled and enjoyed for long enough. Reflect upon the consequences that it has cultivated, and reflect upon all that we've discussed that enables you to take positive action. I'm not sure how much of a dent in this thing I can make but I can assure you that my attempts to sway the fitness of this nation are far from over. Carl Sagan brilliantly stated that the biggest struggle of the 21st century would be to learn how to handle all the advancements we made in the 20th. As we struggle to cope with the advancements and niceties of the 20th century I hope that the 21st can be remembered in history as the great resistance, as the time that we took back control over our fate and moved forward in a new, healthier, and more responsible direction. I hope that in the 22nd century we can look back at these hurdles overcome with reverence and appreciation for the disaster we so forcefully thwarted. This responsibility sits heavy on our shoulders. Yet we have proven before that we are capable of great things and though we've done much to slow ourselves down, I believe we can prove victorious again. We will not go down in history as the once enterprising young species whose fate went down in a gluttonous spiral. So once more I'm asking you to join me. To go forward with Glutton Free Habits, Glutton Free Principles, and a Glutton Free Mind.

Nothing happens to you. Everything happens because of you. Stop blaming, stop complaining. Take extreme ownership of your life and assume responsibility for all your circumstances. Ralph Waldo Emerson said, "The true romance which the world exists to realize is the transformation of genius into practical power."

And remember, don't wish it were easier. Wish you were better.

Don't go Gluten Free, go Glutton Free.

About The Author

As a writer and blogger, Steve Pavel has observed a lot in his 5 short years in the health club industry. As a Health Club Manager and Certified Personal Trainer, Steve Pavel has assisted clients of all types in the world of fitness. He has trained clients in one on one, group, and virtual settings, and is currently working with his team on developing a break through nutrition coaching program to help clients create positive nutrition habits through a habit-based, measured coaching program. You can find Steve's blog on fitness and personal development at GluttonFree.net. As an investor, you can find his blogs on InvestingNoob.com, a website that he has created to help people learn the basics of stock market investing.